THIS BOOK

BELONGS TO

....

....

10 Amazing Benefits Of Using Perfumes

The perfect perfume can boost your confidence just before the big meeting and keep foul body odor at bay. But regularly using perfumes and deodorants benefits you in more ways than smelling great. Floral and fruity scents reduce your stress, give you a morale boost, and help you get the sleep you have been missing out on. In this article, we take a deeper look at the top 10 benefits of using perfumes every day.

Fun Fact

The art of making perfumes, also known as perfumery, was prevalent in the Indus Valley civilization as well as in ancient Egypt and Mesopotamia. Taputti, the first recorded-chemist as per notes on a tablet dating back to 2nd millennium BC in Mesopotamia, is also amongst the first known perfumers.

Benefits Of Using Perfumes

Fragrance

Well, this one is quite obvious. Perfume has been historically used primarily for fragrance. It helps keep unwanted body odor at bay and ensures that you smell good throughout the day.

Enhances Mood

One of the main benefits of wearing perfume is enhancing the mood. Perfume helps lift your spirits. You can also wear a perfume that reflects your mood, to project it better. **Whether you feel playful, mischievous, timid or even reserved, perfumes offer many different kinds of smells for different moods**. Select and wear a perfume as per the occasion so that you can get in the apt mood for it.

Boosts Confidence

Just like a pretty dress, a good perfume can boost your confidence and ensure that you get through the day without feeling conscious of your body odor. A dash of fragrance can work wonders to your **personality.** Choose a scent that suits your personality and which, can boost your morale to fight against all odds.

Makes You Attractive

Sense of smell is one of the most important of the five senses. Sometimes, you can simply get attracted to someone because of the way they smell. Perfumes are rich in pheromones and make you attractive.

Stylecraze Says

Wear warm and invigorating scents such as patchouli, rose, vanilla, cedarwood, bergamot, or sandalwood as these tend to smell soft and animalistic, making you irresistibly attractive when you are going for that vibe.

Aphrodisiac

Many perfumes sometimes function like a natural aphrodisiac. **Certain types of perfumes contain pheromones, which have aphrodisiac properties**. It explains why you get attracted to someone because of their perfume.

Boosts Health

There is no scientific evidence to ascertain the efficacy of perfume's health boosting properties. However, perfume helps enhance the mood, which can keep stress and other anxiety related issues at bay. **You can use your favorite fragrance to beat your anxiety blues and lift your spirits.**

Triggers Memories

Perfume can also be an important trigger of a happy memory. One tends o associate people with particular fragrances. **Many women who wear their mother's signature scent do so to revive memories.**

Try and buy new perfumes every time you travel and wear them. The different perfumes will remind you of each vacation and help you relive those moments.

Aromatherapy

Perfume has many relaxing and therapeutic benefits. Citrus fruit, floral and winter spice perfumes help calm the mind and soothe the body. These perfumes ensure your stress levels are in control.

Treats Insomnia

Another one of the therapeutic effects of perfume is that it helps you sleep better at night. Perfumes, which contain essential oils, can help you relax and enjoy a peaceful slumber at night.

Cures A Headache

This one is a surprise! It is another therapeutic effect of perfume. Wearing a perfume can help you cure that nagging headache. However, this isn't true for perfumes that contain essential oils that compound headache.

Here's Why You Shouldn't Put Perfume on Your Hair – and What to Do Instead

Perhaps you've been stuck in a similar situation before: You're getting ready for the day but haven't shampooed your hair in a few days. You realize that your hair doesn't smell, well, fresh.

You might think that a few spritzes of perfume or body mist on your hair will help, but is it really the best solution?

Not all fragrances are created equal, and your hair deserves tender loving care. Read on to find out what's really the best for stinky hair.

Is it safe?

Technically, it isn't the worst thing you can do to your hair. But it's also not the best. Perfume has the potential to damage your hair.

Consider what ingredients are inside your perfume. Most perfumes and body mists are made with harsh alcohols, like ethyl alcohol, and heavy synthetic fragrances.

According to the Food and Drug Administration (FDA), ethyl alcohol can have a drying effect on skin and hair. For this reason, many cosmetics choose to use other alcohols in their formulas.

Untreated dryness can cause long-term damage, such as breakage, split ends, and frizziness.

Perfume alternatives for hair

There are plenty of perfume alternatives to consider that can maintain the integrity of your hair, cleanse it, and offer hydration.

Hair mists

Consider hair mists as the safest alternative to perfume. These sprays are intended to leave a refreshing, lasting scent without drying out or otherwise damaging your hair.

Shop for hair mists online. Consider these options:

- Infused with a blend of oils, the Sebastian Dark Oil Silkening Mist helps add a natural-looking shine as well as an uplifting scent.

- For a floral scent, try the Aussie Flora Aura Scent Boost Hair Treatment. The formula is lightweight, so you can refresh without compromising your style.

- Prefer something all-natural? The Herbivore Botanicals Hair Perfume Mist scents hair with essential oils and aloe vera.

Dry shampoo

If you're looking for a product that will temporarily clean your hair and add scent at the same time, a dry shampoo is the way to go. These formulas help eliminate excess oils and absorb smells without stripping or damaging hair.

Shop for dry shampoo online. Consider these options:

- Known for its iconic smell, the Amika Perk Up Dry Shampoo deodorizes hair without talc or aluminum.

- With binchotan charcoal, clay, and tapioca, the Briogeo Scalp Revival Dry Shampoo absorbs excess oil while leaving behind a fresh scent.

Scented serums and oils

If you're looking to deeply nourish dry hair, try a scented hair oil or serum. A little goes a long way with these products. You'll probably only need to apply them from the mid-shaft through the ends of your hair.

Shop for serums and oils online. Consider these options:

- The Ouai Hair Oil is a favorite among beauty editors for its lightweight formula that simultaneously protects against heat damage while smoothing out dryness and leaving behind a subtle scent.

- Infused with coconut milk, the OGX Nourishing Coconut Milk Anti-Breakage Serum helps hydrate dry and damaged hair. Plus, it leaves behind a long lasting tropical scent.

Ingredients to look for

While you'll want to stay away from ethyl and isopropyl alcohols, fatty alcohols add hydration and lubrication to hair shafts. Keep your eyes out for formulas with ingredients like:

- cetyl alcohol

- stearyl alcohol

- cetearyl alcohol

These are all derived from plants.

Any hair mists, dry shampoos, or serums that are fortified with natural oils can help repair hair strands and prolong scent.

Essential oils offer an alternative to traditional synthetic fragrances. Just make sure they're safely diluted in a formula to avoid sensitization.

Other things to consider

Avoid cigarette smoke

The smell of cigarette smoke can be absorbed easily into the hair, especially in heavy smokers.

Oftentimes, this is difficult to get rid of and can make hair smell for days.

People who quit smoking typically find that their clothing, hands, and hair stop smelling shortly after.

Wash your hair often

While you might not want to wash your hair every day, sticking to a regular washing routine will ensure better-smelling hair.

This looks different for each person, but many find it best to wash two to three times per week.

You can also use a scalp scrub once a week for a deep clean.

Clean your pillowcase regularly

Wash or switch your pillowcases every week to keep your face and hair clean.

Cotton pillowcases can absorb leftover makeup, bacteria, dirt, and oil, and it all can rub off on hair and skin.

You can also experiment with silk or satin pillowcases. These materials help keep hair from tangling up and further absorbing dirt or oil.

The bottom line

Everyone experiences smelly hair from time to time.

Spraying your favorite perfume on your hair might help short term, but it can damage hair in the long term by drying it out.

For a quick fix, try a formula made for hair, such as a hair mist, dry shampoo, or hair serum.

What to Do About a Perfume Allergy

A perfume or fragrance allergy happens when you have an allergic reaction after being exposed to a perfume that contains an allergen.

Symptoms of a perfume allergy can result from:

- touching the perfume liquid or substance
- getting sprayed by the perfume
- even inhaling some of it

Statistics

According to a 2009 survey on fragrance sensitivity, up to about 30 percent of the population of the United States had irritation from a perfume.

As many as 19 percent of participants in the survey had actual health effects from fragrances.

Perfume allergies are caused in part by over 2,500 chemicals, which are often unlisted, in the average perfume or cologne.

Thanks to laws around "trade secrets" most companies can simply put "fragrance" on their perfumes to represent a hundred or more chemical compounds.

It can be difficult to totally avoid perfumes that cause allergic reactions. But here's some information on:

- what you can do when you notice the symptoms

- how to treat and cope with your allergic reactions

- when to see your doctor

Allergy vs. sensitivity

Allergies

When you have allergies, your body has a specific immune system response to an ingredient or a chemical in the perfume that causes the reaction.

This means that your body identifies the ingredient in the perfume as a foreign substance. Then, it releases an inflammatory reaction to help fight off the substance as if it's a bacterial or viral invader.

This immune system response usually develops over a course of days and manifests as itchiness or a rash. These symptoms can last for weeks before they go away.

Sensitivity

Perfume sensitivity, much more common, is a reaction to something that irritates your body. Sensitivity doesn't necessarily trigger a body-wide immune system response.

With a sensitivity, you might have a rash that goes away after a few hours or a mild headache.

You might also just sneeze a few times before your symptoms go away. This is because your body reacts by getting rid of the irritant to return to normal.

Types of substances

The substance that you react to also makes a difference.

Most ingredients in perfumes that cause a reaction aren't actually allergens. They're usually synthetic or chemical irritants that your body finds… well, irritating.

Allergens, on the other hand, are technically proteins that the body reacts to with an inflammatory response that causes allergy symptoms.

In short, a true perfume allergy happens when an organic protein in a perfume ingredient causes the reaction. The heavy majority of reactions people endure are simply perfume sensitivities.

Symptoms

The symptoms you experience are directly related to whether you have a perfume allergy or a perfume sensitivity.

Let's look at some common symptoms.

Allergy

Most allergic reactions typically give you an itchy red rash that goes away quickly after you've been exposed to the perfume. Some mild symptoms can last for a few weeks even after a brief exposure.

A few mild symptoms of a perfume allergy can include:

- itching, even where you don't see any rash or irritation
- itching around your eyes and in your throat
- skin that's scaly or dry
- blisters that get crusty and ooze pus
- outbreak of hives
- patchy, reddish skin
- a burning sensation on your skin with no visible irritation or sores
- being more sensitive to sunlight than usual

Sensitivity

A few mild symptoms of a perfume sensitivity can include:

- sneezing if the perfume is sprayed near your face and airways (nose, mouth, and throat)
- itching, running, or stuffiness of your nose
- nasal mucus dripping down the back of your throat (postnasal drip)
- persistent cough

- headaches

- nausea

Other allergic reactions are much more severe and can happen quickly. Some of these symptoms might need immediate medical attention. They're however, **extremely** rare.

Here are some severe, emergency symptoms to watch out for:

- **Swelling in your mouth, lips, or tongue.** This kind of swelling can be uncomfortable and make it harder for you to breathe, eat, or talk. You may need medical treatment, such as corticosteroid injections, to reduce the swelling quickly.

- **Anaphylaxis.** Anaphylaxis happens when your airways get inflamed and close up because your body releases a high volume of a type of antibody called IgE. This can make it difficult or impossible to breathe. Get emergency medical help if this happens.

Treatments

Your treatment for a perfume allergy should be based on your symptoms and the substance that causes the allergy.

Most importantly, it should include avoidance of the substance that caused the symptom in the first place.

Try these treatments for mild, temporary symptoms:

- **Medications.** Oral antihistamines like cetirizine (Zyrtec), diphenhydramine (Benadryl), or loratadine (Claritin) can help with itching and stuffiness. You can get these at any store that sells over-the-counter (OTC) medications or get a prescription from your doctor.

- **Topical corticosteroid creams.** You can apply hydrocortisone or other similar steroid creams to an itchy area or to a rash.

- **Colloidal oatmeal bath.** Taking an oatmeal bath can help soothe itching and inflammation. You can also make an oatmeal compress by putting oatmeal soaked in cold water in a thin material like pantyhose.

- **Gentle moisturizing lotion or cream.** Use one that doesn't have any artificial ingredients or chemicals that might trigger another reaction.

- **Try light therapy.** You can try either blue or red light to help eliminate any bacteria irritating your skin or to reduce the immune system response on your skin to both soothe and repair tissue.

If perfume or fragrance allergies are disrupting your life and you want your symptoms to be less severe:

- **Consider getting contact allergen testing.** Your doctor or an allergist can use patch tests that expose you to small amounts of different allergens to determine your specific allergic triggers. Once you figure out what you're allergic to, you can try to avoid any perfumes that contain those ingredients.

Call 911 or seek immediate medical help if you have a fever or any trouble breathing.

How to cope

The first thing you should try to do is avoid the substance causing your allergy in the first place.

Once you know what you're allergic or sensitive to, look for that substance in any perfume you want to buy and never buy it again.

Try natural, plant-based perfumes if you still want to achieve a similar scent but want to avoid any of the substances that cause allergies.

Choosing a perfume that has minimal ingredients can reduce the chance you'll have an allergic or sensitivity reaction.

But you can't always avoid exposure, especially if you live or work with people who wear perfume for personal or professional reasons.

Here are some ways you can help take control of your environment and reduce symptoms of a perfume allergy:

- **Try to avoid common areas** where people wearing perfume may walk by and trigger your allergies or sensitivities.

- Keep a small air purifier near your workspace to help keep your air free of airborne proteins that can trigger your symptoms.

- **Let the people around you know about your allergies**, so they can know to avoid wearing perfume around you.

- **Don't use any scented products at all** to minimize your possible exposure to your allergy or sensitivity triggers. This includes candles and air fresheners.

- **Get a flu shot every year** to keep your immune system strong.

- **Talk to your employer about keeping your workplace scent-free,** especially if you have other coworkers with fragrance allergies or sensitivities.

When to see a doctor

See your doctor as soon as possible if you notice any of the following symptoms:

- large boils or hives that are painful or extremely itchy

- feeling exhausted or drowsy

- feeling confused or disoriented

- feeling unusually dizzy

- feeling sick or throwing up

- heart rate spiking for no reason or beating abnormally

- you have a fever (100.4°F or higher)

- you have symptoms of an infection on your skin or elsewhere, including your skin being warm to the touch or an itchy rash that's producing a thick, cloudy, discolored discharge

- your itchiness or rashes become painfully itchy or constantly distract you from your everyday life

- your rash is spreading out from the place it started to other parts of your body, or new rashes appear where you haven't been exposed

- you have a reaction around your face or your genitals

- **your symptoms don't get any better or start to get** worse after a few days or weeks

- you have trouble breathing because of tightness in your throat

The bottom line

Perfume allergies and sensitivities are common and can be disruptive. This is especially true if you have to work or live with people who wear perfume or cologne every day, and you don't have the ability to avoid them.

But there's plenty you can do to reduce your exposure or improve your symptoms.

Limiting exposure, getting treatment, and telling those around you about your symptoms can help you cope and make sure exposure doesn't interfere with your life.

4 Mistakes To Avoid With Perfume

No, perfume does not cover up smells

The alarm clock has been ringing for a long time, but you hardly get out of bed, no time to take a shower. So, you think that one (or many) sprays will save your day and bring you freshness and cleanliness. We are sorry to disappoint you, but no! Contrary to what Louis XIV and his perfumed court thought, who rarely washed themselves, perfume does not hide bad smells. And above all, it does not make up for the lack of hygiene! Indeed, the perfume will not be able to make you "clean". Worse, the mixture of smells will be all the more dubious! Your colleagues will quickly realize this hazardous technique, and you risk being relegated to the back of the open space…

Taking your deodorant for perfume (or the other way around)

On the other hand, there are those who spray half of their deodorant on their upper body every morning or after a good workout. However, perfume and deodorant are two very different products. While deodorants have sometimes exotic smells, they cannot do the same job as your favorite fragrance. Indeed, the smell of the deodorant, however powerful it may be, will not "perfume" you. The formulas of these two products are very different, and the composition work behind them is even more so. And conversely, perfume does not help you fight perspiration at all.

Don't carry it in your gym bag, it will be lighter (you're welcome). And be careful not to make one of these mistakes by confusing your bottles in the bathroom!

The art of spraying

When you love, you want to enjoy it even more. And you quickly tend to spray the precious scented drops everywhere. Yet there are certain areas of the body that are best suited to enjoy your favorite fragrance even more. We have already told you about it, but do not hesitate to spray your perfume on the "hot" areas of your body. Where smells can weave in and out. These include pulse points such as the neck, the hollow of the knees, the inside of the elbow or the wrists.

Speaking of wrists, one of the biggest mistakes we all make with perfume is rubbing them after spraying. It's not a good idea, and even worse, it makes the skin warm. Enzymes are released and can then slightly modify the smell of your perfume! You can also perfume your hair and clothes, so that the notes follow you even longer.

 "Over-perfuming": not such a good idea

We have already seen it several times, notably, our nose is a formidable appendage with a very powerful memory. And precisely, this olfactory memory stores a very large number of scents in its internal library. Above all, it makes our brain get used to the smells that surround us. From fried food to our perfume, we very quickly have the impression that after a certain time we do not "smell" these odors anymore.

So don't panic! If you have the impression that your perfume does not smell anymore, it's probably because your nose has gotten used to it. But that is not necessarily the case with your neighbors. It is therefore useless to perfume yourself twice as much, at the risk of annoying those around you. Because you should not think that the more perfume you put on, the better you will smell, or the longer the scent will last. "Over-spraying" is therefore rarely pleasant for those who cross your path… And who will keep your scent in their nose for hours on end! Of course, there is no rule about the ideal number of sprays to apply per day. But subtlety and discretion can also be good and can save you from making many mistakes with your perfume.

Contents

Introduction

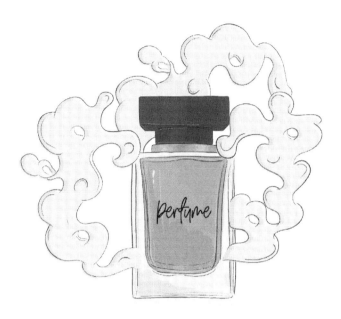

Perfumes make life interesting. Even if you are not in a good mood, the sweet scent of perfume will give you the will to face your day with more energy. A good perfume offers more than just a good smell to your body. It exudes confidence and makes an individual feel special in one way or another. In this book, I am going to show you how to prepare perfumes from natural products such as flowers, tree barks, stems, and other plant matter.

My interest in perfumes started at a tender age. My mother had a wide collection of perfumes, something that attracted interested in their scent. One fine evening, I noticed that the scent my mother was wearing was in every way, similar to the scent of the flowers in our backyard. That is when I decided to find out the relationship between our red roses and the perfume my mother was using. My mother helped me know that perfumes come from flowers; however, she did not explain how. In my stupid mind, I started comparing every perfume I came across to the flowers in my backyard. My obsession with scents and perfumes drove my mother crazy. At some point, she told me never to bother her with questions about flowers and perfumes.

Many years later, I find myself still having an obsession with perfumes. However, my obsession with perfumes today stems from the point of knowledge. I no longer think that every perfume on the shelf is equal to some flowers in my backyard. Years of research have helped me understand the science behind the preparation of perfumes. My obsession with flowers has helped me learn how to prepare perfumes from natural ingredients, including flowers. I have learned that perfumes are much more complex than just a single scent of a single flower. The process of perfume preparation includes scent extractions, scent combination, and scent distribution, among other steps. You cannot just prepare a perfume by picking out the flower that you love and extracting the scent. You will need plenty of special tools, ingredients, and skills.

In this book, I am going to show you the process of preparing perfumes right from the most basic level. Since this is a practical book, we are going to follow the step by step process of preparing various types of perfumes. To ensure that the book is helpful to you, I have broken it into several sections.

In the introductory section of the book, I will introduce you to perfumes. I will help you understand what perfumes are and how they are used. We will also look at some of the terms that are commonly used in the perfumes world. You should expect to encounter some new terms if you are not a botanical or perfume expert. Keep track of these words since they will play an important role in your understanding of the book.

It's important to also keep in mind the fact that we will be using special tools in preparing perfumes. In our second section of the book, I help you shop for the tools needed to prepare perfumes at home. I provide a checklist of tools and materials that are necessary for perfume preparation. There are many methods of perfume preparations, and each method has different requirements. However, if we are going to use botanical extracts, there are specific tools you will need to extract scent from flowers and other natural sources.

In the third section, we get down to business by extracting scent from botanicals. We use diverse methods of extraction to get the scent out of the plants into the perfumes. We prepare tinctures, infusions, and other extracts that are needed. We will not be using plant matter but rather the extracts we prepare when we start preparing perfumes.

In the final section of the book, we get into preparing recipes for perfumes. Whether you love colognes or roll-ons, we have a recipe for you. We prepare two main types of perfumes in our recipes. We focus on liquid perfumes that can be sprayed with a sprayer bottle and solid perfumes such as balms that can be applied in other skincare products.

By purchasing this book, you buy yourself a ticket to the endless world of perfumes. The world of perfumes is vast and with a myriad of scents to choose from. There are thousands of specific scents that you can prepare from independent flowers. This book exploits all varieties of natural products that offer independent scents. Besides the natural products that can offer unique scents, you can also prepare thousands of unique scents by mixing various natural extracts. We will be looking at various ways you can prepare perfumes at home by combining essential oils and natural plant extracts such as tinctures and infusions. In other words, the world of perfumes is very wide and interesting. If you are in love with perfumes, the entire book should be fun for you.

This book is not a case study or a theoretical textbook for students. It is a practical guide, ideal for all those who love perfumes and those who wish to learn to make their own perfumes at home. All the processes in the book are simple and can be done at home. Most importantly, the book provides precautionary measures that all readers must keep in mind to avoid accidents at home. Welcome aboard, and enjoy your reading.

Chapter 1: Introduction to Perfume

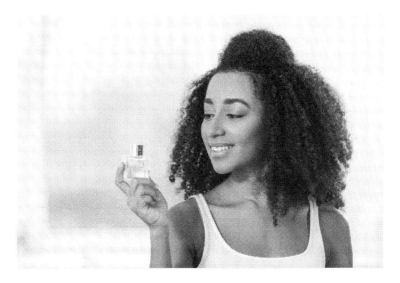

History of Perfume

Before we get down to the details of preparing perfumes, we should get some background information about perfumes. So, where exactly did perfumes originate from? The word perfume originates from a Greek word *perfumare*, meaning "to smoke."

In ancient Greece, perfumes were smoked to provide a sweet scent in religious ceremonies. However, perfumery, the real act of preparing perfumes, started in Mesopotamia, Egypt, India, and China. Evidence shows that perfumery existed in Indus valley civilization as early as 3300BC.

With that said, the documented origin of perfume was in Mesopotamia Egypt. Egyptians used perfumes for various purposes, including beauty and religious ceremonies. The rich elite society of Egypt used perfumes in burial and daily wear. They spent money on expensive perfumes to show their social standings. As it is the case in the modern world, the type of perfume a person wears was used to show their social status in ancient Egypt. However, the practice of perfume making in Egypt remained at a small scale level until the Romans and Greeks learned the art of perfumery. The Romans started producing perfumes in large quantities and standardized quality.

The most tangible evidence of early perfumery was discovered in Cyprus. Scientists unearthed a perfume factory that dates back to 2000BC. The Factory had specialized in producing plant-based perfumes with scents such as coriander, lavender, laurel, and rosemary, among others. Once the Roman Civilization learned how to prepare perfumes, the art started spreading quickly throughout the world. Perfumes were mainly produced for religious purposes during the ancient days. However, in the year 1190, the first commercial perfume industry was established in Paris, France.

How Perfumes are Made

The evolution of the perfume industry has happened over a long time, and the way perfumes are made also evolved. The early Egyptians used to make their perfumes from essential oils. They simply combined balms and ointments with scented essential oils to make perfumes to be applied daily or those used in religious ceremonies.

Today, perfumes are prepared through a much more complex process. A desired quantity of scent is determined and combined with alcohol, such as ethanol or ethanol-water. The concentration of the scent depends on the desired outcome. A true perfume will have a composition of about 40% scent material. However, there are some perfumes where the scent material can be as low as 20%. At the end of the day, the scent material used depends on the final outcome desired.

While in traditional Egypt and the Roman Empire, natural products were used, things have changed today. Most early perfume producers mainly utilized flowers, animals, and seaweed extracted essential oils. Today, the scents that are available in the market do not exist in nature. Synthetic processes such as esterification are used to prepare unique scents that are not available naturally. Most scents today are produced artificially; however, they are often combined with natural scents to provide a natural feel to the perfume.

There are many arguments pitting natural perfumes against artificially produced ones. In this book, we are going to look at some of the ways to prepare perfumes from natural ingredients. However, we will also incorporate some aspects of artificial perfume making.

Glossary of Terms Related to Perfume/Fragrances

To help you understand the book better, here are some of the commonly used terms in the perfume and fragrance world.

Accord: Refers to a combination of notes that are used to produce fragrance in perfume. An accord refers to a combination of two or more ingredients. Notes are the basic building blocks for fragrance. Each perfume is made up of more than one note. One accord might be a combination of two or three notes, while another accord might be a combination of 100 ingredients or more.

Top Notes: This refers to the most prevalent notes in a fragrance. They are what you smell first in perfume. Although an accord might include hundreds of scents, there is the most prevalent scent that you will feel when you encounter the perfume first. This prevalent note is what we refer to as the top note.

Base Notes: This refers to the most tenacious notes in a fragrance. While top notes are instantly felt when you smell the perfume, base notes last longer on your body or clothes when you spray the perfume. Some of the notes that last longer in fragrances include cedar, sandalwood, etc.

Middle Notes: The middle notes are the ones that show up after the top notes disappear. Top notes are felt instantly but quickly vanish. As they vanish, the middle note set in. This category is where you find floral notes. The middle notes of perfume may last for several hours on the skin.

Aromatic: The term aromatic is usually used to refer to anything that has a sweet smell. Aromatic is another word used when referring to perfume ingredients such as lavender, thyme, rosemary flowers, etc.

Compound: This is another name for fragrance, aroma, flavor, or chemical compound. It is a technical term used when referring to scented ingredients used in the preparation of perfumes.

Blend: A blend refers to a mixture of scented ingredients. In the perfume preparation process, we will have to mix various scented compounds to come up with a unique fragrance.

Body: This refers to the heart or the middle part of the fragrance. As we have seen above, a fragrance is made up of top notes, middle notes, and base notes. This is the body of the fragrance.

Cologne: The term cologne was derived from an 18th-century perfume known as *Eau de Cologne*. The term cologne is used when referring to the lightest concentration of perfume. Colognes only has about 2 to 4% of perfume oils and usually lasts2 hours on the skin. While colognes do not last on the skin longer, they are well scented and present a variety of scents for users.

Diffusion: This refers to the process through which perfume travels from the body into the air. Without diffusion, it would not be possible for any person to feel the smell of the perfume.

Distillation: Distillation is a process of extracting scented ingredients from plant material through the use of steam. In the distillation process, the fragrant oils are dissolved in a liquid, which is then heated to separate the solvent from the oils due to their difference in evaporation points.

Eau de Toilette: This is a fragrance that has about 10 to 15% aromatic ingredients. This perfume is prepared by dissolving a base in water or alcohol. This type of fragrance can last up to 3 hours on the skin.

Eau de Parfume: This refers to a perfume with 15 to 20% concentration of aromatic ingredients. This type of perfume can last up to five hours on the skin.

Noses: This is a slang term for a perfumer. Most perfumers do not like this term, but they have to deal with the situation the way it is.

Undertones: This refers to sub characteristics of a fragrance's background that make up the fragrance character.

Balsams: These refer to resins that are rich in oils and smell sweet or soft. Some examples of balsams include Peru balsam, benzoin, tolu, etc.

Citrus: This term is referring to any scent that is citrusy in nature but may also refer to compounds that belong to the citrus family. The most common citrus compounds used in perfume making include lime, lemon, orange, and grapefruit.

Floral: The term floral refers to a fragrance that gives a flowery impression. Most of the perfumes prepared commercially have the middle notes of flowers such as roses, jasmine, lilies, iris, etc. If the fragrance you apply has a noticeable scent of such flowers, it is referred to as being floral.

Musk: This was an ingredient collected from musk deer glands and was used to prepare perfumes. However, fetching musk from deer was outlawed, and now perfume makers have to prepare synthetic musk.

Woody: The term woody refers to a fragrance that evokes the scent of freshly cut wood or dried wood. Some of the ingredients that are used to give perfume a woody scent include vetiver, sandalwood, cedarwood, etc. In most cases, the woody scent is used as a base for the fragrance. It can stay on the skin longer than floral scents.

Gourmand: This refers to a family of fragrances that get their inspiration from the food world. This type of fragrances adopts scents such as chocolate, caramel, vanilla, etc.

Chypre: This refers to a fragrance family that shows sophistication. It includes bergamot and some oakiness within the blend. There are both men and women chypre scents.

Fruity: This refers to fruit notes in a fragrance. In most cases, fruity notes are blended with floral notes. Some of the commonly used fruity notes include blackberry, peach, apple, cherry, or strawberry.

Leather: This refers to a family of fragrance that evokes traditional leather goods scent. In most cases, the leather scent is obtained from compounds such as birch.

Aqueous: These refer to scents that are based on the concept of a watery smell. For instance, a damp piece of wood might have a different smell from a dry one. If the fragrance is inspired by the smell of wet wood, it can be referred to as an aqueous fragrant.

Attar: This refers to fragrant essential oils distilled from flowers. Such types of essential oils are seen as being natural fragrances.

Balsamic: This refers to rich resinous notes produced by using balsams and resins.

Bouquet: This refers to a mixture of flower notes. Most of the fragrances we will be preparing in this book are bouquets since we will mostly use flowers to extract the scent.

Camphoraceous: This refers to the fresh cooling character displayed by eucalyptus and rosemary.

Earthy: The term earthy is used when referring to fragrance notes that give an impression of the soil, forest floor, moss, or mold.

Essential Oil: This refers to the concentrated, volatile aromatic ascent of a plant obtained through distillation. There are many types of essential oils in the market, and each contains special notes.

Evanescent: This refers to perfume notes that are felt quickly and vanish quickly. Most of such notes are used as the top note in most perfumes since they vanish faster.

Extrait (Extract): An alternative name for alcohol-based perfumes. Such perfumes contain about 15 to 45 percent of the perfume compounds in alcohol.

Fixative: This refers to a compound that can be added to perfume to make it last longer. As we have seen, there are some perfumes that do not last past 2 hours on the skin. To make such perfumes last longer, a compound known as fixative is used.

Fougere: These are fragrances based on the herbaceous accord. Such scents may include diverse notes such as lavender, oakmoss, woods, and bergamot.

Green: This is a term used when referring to the odors of greens, such as grass, leaves, and stems.

Leather: This refers to the smokiness characteristics of ingredients that commonly use tanning leather. This scent is achieved in perfumery by the addition of castoreum, labdanum, or some synthetic compounds.

Mossy: This refers to fragrances with an earthy or forest scent.

Oceanic: This refers to perfumes that are scented to evoke natural aromas such as oceanic breeze or mountain air.

Oriental: This refers to a family of fragrance that is based on exotic aromas such as vanilla, oakmoss, and animal notes.

Perfume Defined in Detail

A perfume can be defined as a fragrant liquid made from essential oils, flower extracts, or synthetic compounds. Perfume is used to give a sweet smell to one's body; however, it can also be used for many other purposes. In manufacturing, perfumes are used to give newly manufactured products a certain smell. For instance, perfumes are used to give synthetic leather products a natural leather smell.

The perfumes we are going to prepare in this book will mainly entail mixing alcohol, water, and scented molecules. A smell (scent) simply refers to molecules that are light enough to evaporate at room temperature. Through the diffusion process, molecules easily travel in the air, transferring the sweet smell to all the people in a room. The main reason why alcohol is used in the preparation of perfumes is that alcohol is light and can easily evaporate. This makes it the ideal compound to allow the compounds of any perfume to infuse in a room. Secondly, alcohol also contains esters, which evoke a sweet scent. Depending on the age of fermentation and other factors, different types of alcohol may contain various sweet-smelling esters. These esters help promote the smell of the perfume.

Perfumes are prepared in different strengths. The most concentrated forms of perfumes are perfume oils. Perfume oils are steamed out of the plant or chemically separated. When preparing perfume oils, 98% of alcohol is dissolved in 2% water. This alcoholic mixture is then mixed with alcohol diluted perfume oil. For most of the oil perfumes, the concentration of the scented compound is between 10 % and 45%.

Perfumes are classified according to the scent family. The perfume family mainly refers to the predominant scent in a perfume. For instance, if the primary or dominant scent in a perfume is a certain fruit, such a perfume can be categorized under the fruity family. However, there are no rules followed in grouping the perfumes. In general, perfumes are only grouped based on their smell and are often a concept of common sense.

There are many categories of perfumes, but those that stand out include:

Floral: These are perfumes that smell like flowers. Given that there are diverse types of flowers, there are many brands and types of perfumes that can be classified as floral. In a floral perfume, the top notes represent popularly known flowers and can be felt strongly.

Fruity: The fruity perfumes are the ones that are heavily scented with fruit notes. Just like it is the case with floral perfumes, there is a wide range of fruity perfumes. There are many fruits, and the diversity in fruits also brings diversity in fruit scents.

Green: Green perfumes are those that are prepared from fresh plant matter such as grass or leaves of herbs.

Herbaceous: These are perfumes that are scented with the smell of various herbs. Just like it is the case with the fruity or floral perfumes, there is a diverse range of herbaceous perfumes.

Woody: These are perfumes that have a smell that resembles that of freshly cut wood, dried wood, or wet wood. There are various plants that are used in perfumes to evoke the woody scent. In most cases, woody scented perfumes are more durable since the wood scent stays on the skin longer. In most perfumes, woody scents are used as the base and not the top notes.

Amber: We also have amber perfumes, which are characterized by tree resin scent.

Animalic: We also have animalic perfumes, which are designed to evoke animal smell. Most of these perfumes might evoke a leathery smell of a certain animal, or they may imitate the natural smell of a certain animal.

Musk: These are perfumes that evoke the scent of musk deer. The musk deer fragrance was popular before hunting of these animals was outlawed. Today, musk fragrances are prepared from artificial musk compounds.

Chapter 2: The Basics of Scent and Scent Extraction

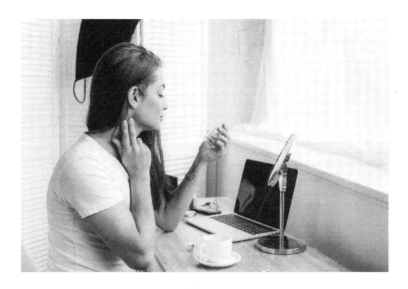

It is a fact that the scent we need to prepare our perfumes is available in nature. Most of the scents we wear are obtained from flowers, roots, and trees, among other natural compounds. However, even though we know that such scents exist, extracting them is not an easy process. Before we even start considering preparing perfumes, we should first look for ways of extracting the scent from plants and other sources.

The first step when you wish to extract scent from flowers or a tree is to collect the natural products you need. If it is flowers, you can purchase fresh flowers from the market, pick yours with a hand from the farm, or order online. The same goes for roots and trunks. You should pick the right roots or stem and cut it into smaller pieces that can be used in your kitchen. Once you have your natural scent material, you will have to purchase the extraction tools. Extraction tools used depend on the extraction process used. In this book, we are going to look at three main methods of extraction. The main methods we will use are enfleurage, solvent, and distillation. These are the methods that were used in ancient days to extract oils from plants and other natural sources. Although these methods are still useful today, we have incorporated modern technology to make the entire process much faster and efficient. Unlike the ancient days where the oils extracted did not have a high concentration of the scent, we can now extract oils that are highly scented.

Tools You Will Need for the Distillation Method

The tools you will need will depend on the process you will be using. For those using all the methods mentioned above, the only method that might require specialized equipment is the distillation method.

Kitchen-size Still: Still refers to a large container that is used in the distillation process. In this process, the flowers or the roots that are supposed to be distilled are added to the still machine, which carries out the rest of the process. A basic still can be purchased on Amazon for as low as $60.

A Steel Tray (to hold the flowers): Some flowers need to be harvested and exposed to the air to give out their full scent. Depending on your source of essential oils, you may be required to have a wide steel tray for air-drying.

A Glass Jar (to store the oil): You will also need a mason jar to store your essential oil once you are done with preparing.

Clean Working Surface: You will also need a clean working surface in an area that does not experience plenty of disruptions. If possible, you should carry your project somewhere else apart from the kitchen

Everyday Utensils: You will also need plenty of other everyday utensils that you already have at home. You should expect to use your knife, some cups, among other common utensils at home.

Tools for the Solvent Process

The solvent process is probably the easiest among all the processes on this list. The solvent process simply involves dissolving the plant matter in natural oils or alcohols. Most of the plant matter can either dissolve or infuse in alcohol. These processes do not need any special equipment, but you should be prepared to bring some tools around.

Solvent Pot: You will need a large glass bottle or a pot where the solvent process will take place.

Cheesecloth: After the plant matter dissolves in your alcohol, you will have to filter it. This calls for fine filtering mediums such as cheesecloth.

Storage Glass Jar: Always have a storage glass jar at hand. Mason jars are the best since they can hold large volumes of the essential oil or tincture extracted.

Common Household Utensils: You might also need some of your everyday household tools. If you are preparing your essential oil in the kitchen, you should not have any problem coming across the necessary tools and materials.

Tools for the Enfleurage

The enfleurage process is another simple way of extracting the beautiful smell from your herbs or flowers. This process simply uses an already existing oil to trap the beautiful scent of the natural source. For this method, you will not need any special tools.

2 Steel Trays: The size of the tray used will depend on the amount of natural material you are going to use in your process. These trays lock the scented flowers in between so that the smell can infuse into your oil.

Plastic Wrap: The plastic wrap will be used to bind the trays together so that they can hold the flowers of plant material in between.

Solid Coconut Oil: We will use solid coconut oil as the medium to tap the scent from the flowers. You can also use any other oil as long as it can trap the scent of the primary material.

Storage Mason Jar: You will definitely need a storage jar for your oil once you are done. The best jar to use is the Mason jar since it does hold sufficient amounts of oil.

Safety Considerations

For all the methods mentioned above, there are various risks involved. You must think about the safety of your family and your personal safety before you even start working. Although each of these methods offers different risks, there are a few general safety guidelines you should observe:

Prepare your extracts away from the reach of children: Children should never come anywhere near your working environment. If you want them to see how the process works, let them observe under supervision. It is only advisable to bring kids around when you are dealing with less risky extraction processes such as enfleurage or the solvent process. However, when it comes to fractional distillation, do not allow children to stay around.

Label all your working equipment if you are working from your kitchen: Some of the processes mentioned here can take as long as a month. If you will be doing the project for that long, you should make sure that all the equipment being used is stored separately from your kitchen tools. Do not use your household utensils in the project and mix them with the other utensils. Always label the utensils that are still being used and keep them aside. Notify all the adult family members about the labeled tools so that they do not end up messing with them.

Wear protective gear: The other general precaution you should take is wearing protective gear. If you are dealing with chemicals or substances that may cause harm to your skin, it is important to wear protective gear. Have your gloves, a pair of glasses, and a face mask if possible. You should also wear your apron if possible, although it is not mandatory.

For still distillation, stay away from flames: The still distillation process involves dissolving your plant matter in alcohol and then distilling it. Given that alcohol is a volatile substance, it can easily lead to a fire outbreak. To avoid the possibility of a fire outbreak, do not smoke or work in an area with open flames. Such flames may lead to an explosion and burn your entire house.

Handle the still pot carefully to avoid getting burned: The still pot gives out a steaming hot gas that may lead to burns if not handled well. Make sure you use a rug when touching any part of your apparatus to avoid getting injured through the process.

Cleaning the Tools and Work Area

Before you start preparing your extracts, you should clean your tools well. You should also clean the tools and the working area after you are done with the work. Given that most of the compounds we will be using in this process are natural, it is important to clean your tools to avoid a case where unwanted bacteria affect the process. It is very critical to clean the tray in the enfleurage process. In this process, we use oils and fresh flowers or roots, both of which can be attacked by foreign bacteria. For the other two methods where we use alcohol, you do not have to worry so much about foreign bacteria. Alcohol is a natural antibacterial and will kill 99% of bacteria and other living matter in your tools.

The first step should always be cleaning with soap and water. Clean your tools with the normal bar soap and rinse with water. However, this only applies to solid washable tools. Once they are clean, rinse them in flowing water for over 1 minute. Place the tools on a dish rack and let them dry naturally before use.

For the still, you have to wash immediately after use. If you let the pot stay with the dirt, you may never be able to clean it in the future. To clean your still, fill the pot to about 20% with a mixture of white vinegar and distilled water in the ratio of 1:1. This means that you combine 50% water with 50% white vinegar. Preheat your still and run through the water and vinegar mixture above. Cut the water and rinse your still with clean water. Discharge the water and heat for about 30 seconds to dry it off.

How to Prepare Botanicals

If you have ever brewed a cup of tea at home, you have already prepared a botanical at home, even without knowing. Some botanicals are as easy and simple to make as a cup of tea, while others are more tedious and complex.

The term *botanical* simply refers to any substance that is extracted from plants. When we talk about perfumes, a botanical is a plant extract that is prepared with the purpose of giving out a specific scent. Most of the perfumes you purchased in the store contain some amount of botanicals. If you love flowers, you have probably come across all sorts of scents, some of which are easily identified in perfume brands available in the market.

In this section, we are going to focus on extracting the scent from various plants. The process of extraction depends on which plant you are dealing with and the type of extract you hope to end up with. As we have already seen above, you can dissolve, diffuse, or distill to the extract. In this section, I want us to focus on the extracts that are the easiest to prepare at home. As you can see from our list of tools in the sections above, some of the items you may need are not readily available at home. However, by purchasing the mentioned tools, you should be ready to prepare your botanicals. We are going to classify our botanicals into 3 main categories; tinctures, extracts, and infusions.

Tinctures, Extracts, and Infusions

Most people assume that the words tincture, extract, and infusion mean the same thing. In reality, they are very different types of botanicals. Although they all contain compounds extracted from plant material, they do not resemble each other in composition or looks.

The first point you should take home is that tinctures and extracts are prepared through an infusion. In other words, tinctures and extracts are just infusions except that they have different concentrations of the plant matter. The process of extracting chemical compounds from a plant is what we refer to as infusion. There are many ways of infusion, and the method you use will determine whether you end up with an extract, tincture, or simply an infusion.

As to whether the final product is referred to as an infusion, an extract, or a tincture depends on the concentration of the plant matter. For instance, in the case where the plant is being infused in alcohol or glycerin, it is likely to end up in a tincture or an extract. An extract is an infusion where the final product is 1 part herb to 1 part alcohol. In other words, the ratio of alcohol to herb is 1:1. This is a very strong product and will offer the best scent for those seeking to extract the valuable scent of the plant. On the other hand, a tincture is considered 1 part herb to 3 parts of alcohol. This shows that a tincture contains more alcohol or glycerin than it contains the herb. The plant to alcohol ratio, in this case, will be 1:3.

If you wish to extract the valuable chemicals out of any plant matter, it is advisable to pick the delicate ones. This would mean that it is better to pick the leaves or flowers. However, since some of the scents we need may be hidden in the stem of roots, we infuse any part of the plant for the purposes of extracting scent. If you wish to have an oak woody smell, you will have to infuse the bark of an oak tree. This will ensure that you get the oaky smell in your infusion, which can then be used in preparing your perfumes.

There are many methods of infusion, although most of them use similar ingredients. The main ingredients used in infusion are hydrocarbons- either alcohol or oils. Most people use ethanol or glycerin. With that said, other ingredients can also be used for infusion purposes. However, since our aim is to extract scent, we are going to use methods that allow you to extract essential oils. It is only through extracting essential oils that you are in a position to capture scented trichomes that are needed in perfume preparations. We have hot and cold infusions as the main methods of infusion used at home. The method you choose depends on the type of plant being infused and how much of the extract you wish to extract.

Hot Infusions: Hot infusion is the ideal process to bring out the chemical compounds of any plant. The infusion brings out vitamins, enzymes, and essential oils with aromatic notes. Our interest is to capture the aromatic notes through the essential oils. However, this method can be harsh on some aspects of the plant. If the scent of the plant is volatile, chances are that you may lose the scent in the heating process. Therefore, there are some plants that are well suited for hot infusion, while others are not. I will recommend using hot infusion when dealing with the least delicate parts of a plant. For instance, if you have to extract aromatic notes from the stem of a tree or its roots, the best option is to use the hot infusion. On the other hand, if you wish to extract scent notes from the leaves or flowers, cold infusion would be okay.

Cold Infusions: The cold infusion process works well for plants that are heat sensitive. In other words, if the plant loses its important ingredients when exposed to heat, you should opt for cold infusion. The tender parts of most plants are ready to release the important chemical compounds without the need to heat. When we use flowers or leaves, it is advisable to stick to cold infusion, unless you are dealing with a plant that is known to be inherently stubborn in releasing its compounds.

How to Prepare a Tincture

Tinctures present the perfect way of extracting scent notes for your perfumes. The reason why I recommend tinctures is that most tinctures are prepared with alcohol. Although a tincture can be prepared with vinegar or glycerin, you should stick to alcohol if you are preparing your tinctures for the purpose of extracting scent notes. Normally, vinegar and glycerin come with other aromas that may affect the scent of your plant matter. Alcohol is the best option because we will also be using alcohol in preparing perfumes. As we have already mentioned, most perfumes contain at least 50% alcohol. In other words, just by infusing your plant matter into high proof alcohol, you are likely to end up with a basic perfume to use at home. Here is the process of preparing tinctures from any type of plant at home.

What you need:

Herbs of your choice (choose the part of the plant with the strongest smell)

40% vodka, clear

1 glass jar

Parchment paper

Masking tape for labeling

Cheesecloth

Directions:

1. Fill up your glass jar to the halfway mark with your preferred herbs. If they are in large chunks, cut them into small pieces to increase the surface area for infusion.

2. Now add your clear, 80 proof alcohol such that the liquid is 2' inches or more above the herbs. If you are using dried herbs, you might have to add in more vodka later.

3. Now place a parchment paper between the lid and jar and tighten the lid. The parchment paper is important since it helps prevent the lid from dissolving in the alcohol.

4. Label your jar with a date and time and shake vigorously. Keep your jar in a cool dark place and shake two times each day for 1 month.

5. After 1 month, strain the resulting tincture through cheesecloth and discard the plant matter

6. Store your tincture in a dark glass bottle in a cool dark place until time for use. The tincture prepared in this process should contain

sufficient herb scent for your project. As you open the jar for straining, you should feel a strong smell of the herb scent emanating from the tincture.

If you were using sweet-smelling flowers such as roses, you might as well apply the tincture to your skin directly. However, this tincture should only be used with other combinations to prepare your preferred perfume.

How to Prepare an Infusion

As already mentioned, there are two types of infusion. We have hot and cold infusions. You can either infuse the scent of your flowers in water, oil, or alcohol. In this recipe, I am going to show you how to infuse the scent of your herbs into the water using both the hot and cold process.

What you will need:

Herbs of your choice (dried herbs work better if they still contain the aroma you are looking for)

Boiling water

Directions:

1. Scoop about 3 tablespoons of dried herbs into a glass jar or use fresh leaves in an equal measure.

2. Pour 1 cup of hot boiling water over your herbs and tighten the lid.

3. Let your herbs steep in hot water for about 30 minutes to release the valuable aromatic chemicals.

4. Strain the herbs out using cheesecloth and store water in a clean dark glass for later use.

If you inhale the vapor from the water, you should smell the aromatic aspects of the plant. With this process, you can also infuse using other types of liquids, such as oil and alcohol. However, you should be careful when heating alcohol since it can easily evaporate.

Cold Process Infusion

1. Fill a quart jar with cold water.

2. Wrap 1 ounce of your preferred herbs in cheesecloth. To ensure that the herbs mix well with your water, lightly moisten them before wrapping the cheesecloth.

3. Submerge your herbs just below the water in your jar and tighten the lid. To ensure that the cheesecloth does not drop to the bottom of your jar, drape the tied end of the bundle over the lip of the jar.

4. Secure by loosely screwing the cap and let the herbs infuse overnight. You may refrigerate for more effective infusion.

5. After about 12 hours of infusion, remove the cheesecloth from your water and store your scented herbal water in a dark glass until time for use.

Alternative Cold Process Infusion

Although the cheesecloth method is the best option for infusion, it does not allow the herbs to infuse effectively. The only reason this method is preferred is that it does not allow any plant matter to remain within the final infusion. The other option we can use when infusing our plant matter into water is the direct method. In this method, the plant matter is directly submerged in the cold water and allowed to infuse overnight.

1. Place your chopped herbs in a quart jar.

2. Top up with water until it is at least 2 inches over the herbs.

3. Allow the herbs to infuse in a cool place or refrigerate for a more effective outcome.

4. After about 12 hours of infusion, strain out the plant matter with cheesecloth and store your aromatic infusion in a dark glass bottle.

How Distillation Works

Essential oils are the most common type of perfumery oil. Essential oils offer the strongest scent of the original plant because they are extracted with all the aromatic trichomes. The best way of extracting aromatic compounds in any plant is by extracting essential oils. For all our perfume preparations, we will focus on combining various essential oils with other extracts such as tinctures and infusions.

Distillation is the best-known process of separating essential oils from the plant. When plants are heated, the essential oils escape through the steam. The steam is then collected through condensation. This is the process we refer to as distillation. There are various types of distillation, as we will see. While distillation offers the best option for extracting aromatic compounds from plants, there are various challenges that make it impractical for home-distillers. At a local level, distillation is possible, although it comes at a much higher cost than the other methods of extraction discussed above. However, the best distillation is practiced by commercial producers of essential oils. You either have the option of purchasing essential oils for your perfumery projects, or you could decide to extract yours at home. In the industrial extraction of essential oils, the CO_2 extraction method is the most effective. In CO_2 extraction, a supercritical fluid is blasted through the plant-extracting the volatile plant material. The volatile plant materials are then collected as essential oils and are used in preparing perfumes.

This type of distillation is more expensive than traditional methods of distillation and cannot be used at home. However, it is the most effective way of distillation, and it offers the highest quality of essential oils.

Dry Distillation

For those of you who wish to obtain some aromatic substances but cannot afford CO_2 distillation, there are other options. You can either use dry distillation, or you may use fractional distillation. The dry distillation method is a process that happens naturally, and you do not have to take any action to separate the aromatic trichomes from the plant. In dry distillation, what we harvest is known as resin. Resins are the often sticky substances found on tree barks. Resins were traditionally burned as incense or offered to gods. Today, these substances that are extracted naturally can be harvested and used to spice up your perfume. The beauty of resins is that they form the base notes of the perfume, and they stay longer on the skin than the floral or fruity smells. Today, resins are used to offer smoky, woody, and amber notes to the perfume. Some of the common resins available in the market today include frankincense, myrrh, and fir. They are either gum resins or hard resins that can be harvested from the bark of trees such as oak.

There are various ways of harvesting these important notes from the bark of a tree. You can either tap into the bark of the tree or collect the resins in a glass jar if they are available in sufficient amounts. You can also obtain the resins through the steam distillation process described above.

Fractional Distillation

The most common and easiest type of distillation is fractional distillation. Fractional distillation is similar to CO_2 extraction, except that you do not have to use supercritical fluid. Heating your plant matter in your kitchen can help you distill the important aromatic trichomes out of the plant. In our equipment section above, we have mentioned that you will need a still to distill your flowers. The still pot offers the best and easiest way to distill the aromatic substances out of your plant material. The fractional distillation process can easily be fulfilled at home if you have a still and some alcohol.

What you need:

Pot still

80 proof alcohol

Preferred herbs

Directions:

Combine your preferred herbs with the alcohol in your still and turn it on.

The alcohol will heat up to a supercritical point and evaporate, picking some of the important elements of the plant. The alcohol is then collected in the condensation chamber. The alcohol will contain high volumes of essential oil, which can be further evaporated to remain with pure essential oil.

Understanding Enfleurage

The other process of extracting trichomes from your herbs is enfleurage. This is a way of extracting the fragrance of the plant by exposing it to odorless fats at room temperature. While there are no fats that are completely odorless, there are those that do not have a strong smell. If you wish to extract the sweet scent of iris, you can simply expose them to any odorless fat at room temperature.

What you will need:

Solid odorless coconut oil at room temperature

Two steel trays large enough to hold your plant matter in a thin layer

Plastic wrap

Directions:

1. Using your hands, spread the solid oil on the surface of one tray to make a thin layer.

2. Once you have a thin solid layer on your tray, spread your herbs over the solid fat such that it covers all the oil. This process works well if you are using leaves or flowers.

3. Once they form a thin layer above the oil, place the second steel tray over the first tray and press it such that it pushes the herbs into the oil in the first tray.

4. Using your plastic wrap, tightly hold the two trays together such that there is no space in between them.

5. Place your trays in a cool, dry place and let them stay there for about 48 hours.

6. After 48 hours, remove the top tray and gently pick out the plant matter. Make sure you do not pick any of the oil from the tray.

7. Once you have removed all the plant matter, warm your coconut oil over low heat so that it melts.

8. Transfer the oil into a clean Mason jar and store it in a cool dark place until time for use.

If you have used flower petals from any of your favorite plants, the oil should have a strong scent of your flowers. You may also combine various flowers if you wish to combine their smell in a single oil.

How to Store Tinctures, Distillates, and Infusions

Tinctures, distillates, and infusions are just herbs stored in different forms. As you can see from the sections above, we prepare these extracts by either dissolving the herbs in water, alcohol, or oil. The solvent used affects the shelf life of the herbs in one way or another. There are various ways that such extracts can get spoiled. First, if the infusion is attacked by bacteria, it will start decomposing. The other option would be the infusion going rancid. Here are some guidelines to observe when dealing with infusions.

Water-based Infusions

Water-based infusions are the most vulnerable to bacterial attacks. Such infusions will easily go bad if you do not store them properly. Water-based infusions usually have a shelf life of about 24 hours. This specifically applies to cold infusions.

Any product that is prepared through the cold infusion process shown above will have a very short shelf life. Most of such extracts will only remain fresh and retain the sweet smell within 24 hours. On the other hand, if your extract is prepared through steam hydrolysis, it will have a shelf life of up to 24 months. However, this is also subject to the botanical used in the process.

There are some herbs that naturally have a higher pH than others. If a plant has a higher pH, it is likely to go bad faster than those with lower pH. The rate at which bacteria attack certain extracts depends on the level of acidity. High acidity reduces the risk of bacterial infection in any organic matter.

With that said, it is important to keep in mind the fact that the main reason why we are preparing these infusions is to capture the aroma of the plants. The aroma captured cannot stay in your extracts for a very long time. It is, therefore, necessary to use your infusions as soon as possible. To ensure that the aroma does not escape, always store your water-based infusion in a dark glass bottle and tighten the lid.

While the actual shelf life of most water-based infusions might be less than 24 hours, the lifespan of such products can be increased by refrigeration. By refrigerating water-based infusion, you can have them around for several weeks without having to worry about them going rancid.

Oil-based Infusions

The shelf life of oil-based infusions is much longer than that of water-based infusions. While oil can stay for a considerably long time without getting infected by bacteria, the organic herbs in the oil can lead to rancidity. The shelf life of most oil-based infusions is between 6 months and 3 years. There are some oils that are easily oxidized when exposed to air. If you happen to use oil that oxidizes easily, just add an antioxidant product like vitamin E or rosemary oil the extract to improve its lifespan.

With all that said, you may also increase the lifespan of your oil-based infusions by refrigeration. Just refrigerate the extract in your glass jar for a lifespan of between 12 months and 5 years. However, most of the products we have prepared should be used within 1 year of preparation. While infusions may have a very long lifespan, the aromatic compounds in the infusion are better used while they are still very active. This should be within 6 to 12 months of infusion.

Alcohol-based Infusions

Alcohol-based infusions such as tinctures tend to have the longest shelf life. Alcohol is a natural antibacterial, which means that it protects the tincture from the possible bacterial attack. This is another reason why you should opt for alcohol when preparing your tinctures as opposed to using glycerin or vinegar.

Most tinctures have a lifespan of between 3 to 5 years. However, if you want your tincture to have a long shelf life of at least three years, you will have to use high proof alcohol. For example, the tincture recipe above shows you the way to prepare a botanical extract with an 80 proof vodka. This means that the vodka used is 40% pure alcohol. This type of tincture can last up to 5 years without being refrigerated. Further, if the alcohol is kept in a dark place in a glass bottle, it will not get oxidized.

It's also important to ensure that before you store your tincture, it is well filtered. Any plant matter that remains in your tincture may attract bacteria that may lead to the tincture going bad.

Vinegar-based Infusions

Although we have not prepared any vinegar-based infusions, they are among the most commonly used infusions. Vinegar can be used in a similar way as alcohol in preparing tinctures. While vinegar will extract the scent you need from your plant, it might affect the smell since it has a pungent smell. If you choose to use vinegar, choose one that does not have a strong smell.

Any Product made from vinegar with more than 5% of vinegar should have a shelf life of at least 6 months. This also depends on the nature of the plant used. Some plants have a lower pH than others, and that might affect the overall shelf life of your tincture. Just like it is the case with alcohol-based tinctures, vinegar-based infusions should be well filtered. Leaving any plant-based matter in your tincture will accelerate the rate of bacterial infection. You may also refrigerate your tinctures for a much longer lifespan.

Dried Herbs/Resin Storage

Lastly, you can also extract resin from the barks of trees, as we have seen in the dry distillation process above. You may also obtain dry extracts by completely evaporating the water after infusing your herbs in water or alcohol. The only dry herb extract with a long lifespan is dry resin harvested from the bark of trees. However, if you evaporate water from your infusions, the dry extracts obtained will have a reduced life span. Any dry extract obtained through other methods other than the resin collected from tree barks will have a shorter lifespan. Generally, it is recommended to use your powdered extracts within 6 to 12 months of preparation.

Understanding Essential Oils

Essential oils are volatile oils that are found in many plants. Almost all types of plants contain essential oils. These oils are different from fatty oils because they evaporate on contact with air. In other words, as soon as essential oils are exposed to air, they start diffusing. The main reason why we harvest essential oils for perfume preparation is that they are harvested with the aromatic compounds in every plant. As we have seen from the distillation processes above, most essential oils are harvested for the purpose of the pleasant aromatic notes of the plant. Given that essential oils evaporate when they are exposed to air, you will feel the strong smell of any plant from the essential oil after harvesting it.

Essential oils can be harvested through any of the methods discussed above. The infusion techniques we have looked at can harvest the oil and the aromatic notes in any plant; however, the strength of the aroma is very weak. In most cases, the aromatic notes will not be felt as strongly as you may experience in a perfume purchased off the shelf. While we may have a desire to prepare perfumes from natural products, we should also strive to prepare a perfume that is sweet-scented and one that adds value to your fashion. There is no point in wearing a perfume that is barely noticeable.

Most people who choose to prepare perfumes at home have the option of either extracting essential oils or purchasing oils that have already been prepared. If you choose to prepare your essential oils at home, I will recommend using the distillation method. Distillation will provide the highest quality oil that can be used in all your recipes. With that said, most of our recipes will require a combination of more than 1 type of essential oil. If you will be using several types of oil to prepare your perfume, you will need to have plenty of time to prepare diverse types of oils for your project.

If you do not have time to prepare diverse types of oil, you will have to purchase the essential oils for your project. As a matter of fact, it is recommended that you purchase your oils from the market if you are looking to get the strongest scent. Commercial producers have the tools that are needed to produce pure essential oils with the strongest scent. If you have purchased any type of essential oil before, you can testify that they are strongly scented. Such oils are readily available in most stores and online shops. You can actually purchase any type of essential oil, including those made from flowers, stems, and roots, from online stores. Most of these oils have a very strong scent and can help you prepare the best perfumes out there.

How to Construct a Specific Scent

It is possible for any person to construct a specific scent. As we have already seen, every scent is made up of various notes. For instance, a single scent might be made up of fruity and woody notes. Any complete scent should be made up of at least 3 notes. We should have the top note, the middle note, and the base notes.

If you are out to construct a specific scent, you should start by choosing the base notes you wish to have in your perfume. As already mentioned, we are going to use essential oils to prepare most of our perfumes. Pure essential oils are the perfect choice for any person who is looking to utilize independent notes. For instance, lavender oil will have floral notes that are related to the lavender flower. If you wish your unique scent to have a lavender feel, you should ensure that lavender essential oil is part of your notes.

As to whether an essential oil is classified as being among the top, middle, or base notes depends on its rate of diffusion. The essential oils that diffuse faster and disappear quickly are often classified as top notes. Those that diffuse moderately and take some time to disappear are classified as middle notes, while those that diffuse slowly and last the longest are referred to as base notes. Here are some classifications of essential oils in terms of notes.

Base Notes: Base notes are mostly essential oils extracted from tree barks. Such oils do not diffuse as fast as those harvested from flowers. They form the base of the fragrance and will remain on the skin longest. Some essential oils that can be classified as base notes include cedarwood, cinnamon, sandalwood, neroli, and nutmeg, among others.

Middle Notes: These are mainly essential oils that do not diffuse very fast, but they do not last long either. When you open a perfume, the first smell to hit your nose is the top notes. After a short while, you will start experiencing the middle notes. Some of the essential oils that can be used as middle notes include clove, lemongrass, geranium, lime, lemon, orchid, etc.

Top Notes: The top notes are made up of the most volatile scents. If you are using essential oils, some of the most volatile oils that can act as your top notes include lavender, jasmine, roses, orchids, etc.

Bridge Notes: With the tree notes above, you are ready to develop your own unique scent. However, you may also want to include bridging notes. These are scents that can appear in between the three notes above. If you are using essential oils, some of the bridging notes you can use include vanilla and lavender.

Once you have all the essential oils, you need to find a compound that will combine all these notes together. As we have already discussed, nothing works better than alcohol. Most perfumes are made up of at least 50% alcohol. However, if you are just trying to come up with a unique scent for the first time, you could use as much as 90% alcohol and reserve your essential oils to 10% or less.

From the list of essential oils with specific notes above, choose the ones you want to appear as your base notes, the middle notes, and the top notes. You should also remember that the smell of your specific ascent will be changing with time. If you wish your fragrance to stay on the skin longer, choose a strong base note such as cedarwood essential oil. With these few ingredients, you are ready to come up with your own unique scent. I am going to show you the full recipes on how to prepare your unique perfumes in the following chapters.

Chapter 3: Understanding the Science of Perfume

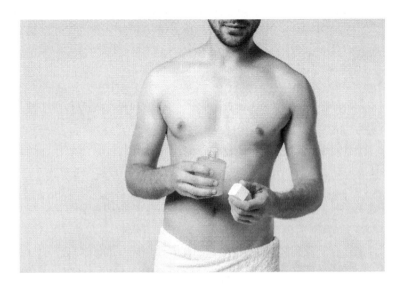

Perfume production is an old tradition. As we have seen in the history section, people started producing perfumes as early as 3000BC. While the art of perfume production has been around for a very long time, there have been several changes in the art of perfume production throughout the years. Early perfume producers mainly relied on natural products, while modern producers have diverse ways of producing perfumes. At the same time, alcohol was introduced into perfume production, replacing the traditional practice where oils were used. In this chapter, we are going to look at the basic principles that guide perfume making. We will determine the exact steps that are taken in manufacturing perfumes and how you can implement these steps at home.

Basic Steps in Making Perfume

While each perfume has a different method of making, there is a general approach used when making perfumes. Just like it is the case with baking bread, there are obvious steps that you cannot skip when making perfume. Among the important steps include the extraction of scent from natural products, blending of scents, and aging, among others. If you are interested in making perfume, you must learn how to follow these steps to ensure that you end up with a well-scented perfume. Here are the main steps involved in perfume making.

Step 1: Extracting essential oils from natural products.

The first and the most important step in perfume making is extracting essential oils from natural products. As we have already seen in the chapters above, you will need three scent notes to prepare your perfume. The natural products you use should be able to give you the three basic notes that make up the perfume. Top notes can be acquired from highly scented flowers such as roses or lavender. Middle notes can be obtained from moderately scented plants or flowers such as iris, lemongrass, or lime. The base notes are often obtained from tree barks such as cedar, oak, etc.

Before you settle down to start making your perfume, make sure you extract at least three essential oils with each of the oils representing at least one of the notes. There are many methods of extracting essential oils, as we have already discussed above. You can either use the infusion, solvent, enfleurage, or distillation method. The most effective method of extracting essential oils from a plant is distillation. Distillation allows you to extract pure essential oils that are rich in pure scent from the plant of your desire.

Besides the essential oils used in preparing perfumes, there are other products that need to be collected. For instance, some perfumes use deer musk in the recipe. If you cannot access deer musk, you can purchase synthetic musk from the market. Lastly, ensure that you have the blending ingredient around. For most perfumes, alcohol is used as the blending ingredient. If you are going to blend your perfumes with alcohol, use at least 80% proof alcohol for the project. You can use clear alcohol to avoid preparing a perfume that will stain your clothes. You may also use amber or golden colored vodka as long as the portion of alcohol used in the recipe is limited.

Step 2: Blending the Ingredients

Once you are done with extracting the essential oils from natural products, you can move to the next step, which simply involves blending your essential oils. As mentioned, it is important to consider the required notes when extracting your essential oils. The essential oils extracted are then blended according to a predetermined formula. The formula you use depends on the desired final outcome. If you are aiming to attain a predetermined scent, you will have to follow a specific formula set by experts in the perfume industry.

For instance, if you have to prepare a perfume that resembles a known brand in the market, you will have to get the exact formula used by that brand. On the other hand, if you wish to prepare perfume that is unique and a scent that represents your interests, you can come up with your own formula. Arriving at the right perfume formula is not easy either. If you wish to come up with your own unique scent, you will have to go through a long trial and error process. In other words, you will have to try blending several recipes until you arrive at one that gives you your desired smell.

Step 3: The Aging Process

Most high-quality perfumes have to undergo an aging process. Some of the premium perfumes purchased in the market have to undergo several months of aging and some even years. When the blended perfumes are aged, the perfect scent is created. By combining essential oils, you do not create the required scent. It is the time taken to age the perfumes within the right environment that gives them their scent. In some cases, base notes are infused into the perfume during the aging process.

Quality Control

Finally, the perfume produced has to undergo quality control. Quality control is simply a process of determining whether the final product is fit for the consumers. In most cases, quality control involves testing the product at an individual level and at a governmental level. At an individual level, you can test the quality of the perfume prepared by spraying it on yourself. When testing the quality of your perfume, you will have to check it against some set standards.

First, test to see whether the perfume prepared meets your intended scent. If it meets your intended scent, you should experience the top notes as anticipated; similarly, you should also experience the middle and base notes afterward. Secondly, you should test the duration that the perfume takes to fade away. As we have discussed, colognes can vanish from the skin in 2 hours. At the same time, there are some perfumes that can last more than 5 hours on the skin. You should test your perfume to determine how long it stays on your skin after application.

The other aspect you should test for is the effect of the perfume on your body and on other people around. There are people who are allergic to specific smells. You should test to see if anyone around you gets affected by the scent of your perfume.

With that said, the actual work of quality control is carried out by government institutions set to test the quality of products. If you are producing your perfume for commercial purposes, you must submit samples to government officials to get a clear picture of the quality of the product you have prepared.

Using Fresh Elements in the Perfume

Fresh elements can be used in all types of perfumes, whether your perfume is synthetic or natural. For those who wish to prepare natural perfumes, it is very easy to add fresh element scents into your perfume without necessarily adding the oil from these fresh elements. In general, there are 4 ways of adding fresh elements into perfume.

1. Prepare essential oil with your elements: The most appropriate way of adding natural elements to your perfume is by preparing essential oils. As you can see from the process above, preparing any perfume is simply a combination of various essential oils. However, commercial perfume manufacturers attain diverse scents by introducing synthetic scents that may not be available in nature. For the purpose of this book, we will mainly focus on scents that are already available in nature. As a matter of fact, most of the perfume scents used in industrial production are available in nature. If you wish to have any natural fresh product smell in your perfume, just use the product to make your essential oil. Use the essential oil prepared in your oil making formula to attain an oil that is made with fresh elements.

2. Infuse the elements into the essential oils: The other option you have is to infuse the fresh elements into essential oils. For instance, if you wish to prepare a perfume with some notes of lavender, yet you do not have access to lavender essential oil, you can simply infuse lavender in your essential oil. Let's say you have olive oil as one of the essential oils you are going to use in your recipe. You can simply infuse your lavender into the olive oil and have a strong smell of fresh lavender in your olive essential oil.

The process of infusing any fresh element is as simple as the process of infusion discussed in the chapter above. For instance, if you wish to infuse lavender scent into your olive oil, all you have to do is add lavender flowers in your oil and let them stay in the refrigerator for about 24 hours. After 24 hours, remove your olive oil from the refrigerator and use it in preparing your perfume in combination with other essential oils of your choice. In this process, you will end up having notes of lavender in your perfume, even if you do not use lavender essential oil. However, this approach should only be used when extracting middle notes and bridging notes. You cannot extract top notes or base notes with this approach.

3. Age the perfume with fresh elements: The other option is to age your perfume with fresh elements. Once your perfume is prepared, it has to undergo an aging process. If the aging process is about 6 months, you can infuse the required fresh elements in the perfume during this period. For instance, if you want to have the cedarwood scent in your perfume but do not have access to cedar oil in any form, you could age your perfume with cedar chips. Just like we did with lavender infusion in the stages above, you will have to add cedar chips in the perfume to be aged. Lock the woods in your perfume and let them stay within the perfume throughout the aging process. If you are aiming at extracting the cedarwood scent, you must be clear about the type of cedarwood scent you wish to extract. If you are aiming at dried cedarwood scent, use the dried chip. If you wish to have a fresh cedarwood smell, use fresh cedar wood chips. The same can be applied to other fresh elements, including flowers. However, you should keep in mind that some fresh elements could contaminate your perfumes if they are left to stay for too long. For instance, if your perfume has an aging period of 1 year, and you want to infuse fresh lavender in it, do not allow the flowers to stay in your perfume throughout the aging period. You could remove the leaves after 1 month and allow the perfume to continue with the aging period.

4. Add fresh elements directly: The other way of adding fresh elements into your perfume is by directly mixing the fresh element with your perfume. Although this approach is not recommended, there are some fresh products that can easily be mixed with perfume. For example, if you wish to have a citrus scent in your perfume and you do not use any citrus-scented oils, you can directly add some lemon juice to your perfume. Just squeeze sufficient lemon juice out of fresh lemon and mix it with your perfume before the aging period. Once well mixed, age your perfume accordingly. There are many fruits that can be squeezed to give out the juice that can be mixed with the perfume. However, you should be careful not to mix your perfume with colored fruit juices. Such juices may dirty your clothes when you are spraying your perfume.

Incorporating Essential Oils in Your Perfume

As mentioned, essential oils are the most basic building blocks for most perfumes. In other words, it is almost impossible to come up with any natural perfume without using essential oils. As we have seen in our oil preparation formula above, you need to extract essential oils first and combine them with other essential oils to come up with your preferred scent. With that said, there is a procedure that should be followed when incorporating your essential oils into perfumes. You can either mix essential oils when blending a fresh scent, or you may incorporate essential oils in an already existing perfume. In either case, there are procedures that should be followed to ensure that the essential oil offers the right scent.

Mixing Essential Oils in an Existing Perfume

The process of mixing essential oil in an already existing perfume is very different from the process of developing a fresh blend. However, if you do not want to undergo the hard work of building a fresh blend from scratch, you can use this option. There are very many types of industrial perfumes out there that can be improved by the addition of essential oils. Some of the colognes that last for 2 hours on the skin can be made to last longer by adding some essential oils. However, the process of adding essential oils is never easy. If you are going to mix an essential oil in an already existing perfume, you should follow these steps:

Determine the perfect scent to add: The first step should be determining the right scent to add to your perfume. If you are trying to incorporate a fresh scent into an already prepared perfume, target adding either a middle or base note. Middle notes offer the best option because they are less dominant. Adding an extra top note to your perfume might end up messing with the entire scent of the perfume.

Determine the ratio of addition: The hardest part about adding essential oil to an already existing perfume is coming up with the right ratio. To determine the ratio of the new essential oil, you must first determine the original formula used in preparing the perfume. Once you determine the formula, you may have to increase the volume of the other essential oils in the perfume before adding your new scent. For instance, if the perfume had lavender essential oil as the top note and nutmeg as the middle note, you would have to determine their ratios first. If you wish to introduce I rose essential oil as the middle note, it should not overpower the scent of the other scents in the perfume. Make sure it balances to ensure that your new perfume is well balanced.

Mix well and give it time to age: Once you have found the right ratio, mix your essential oil with the perfume and give it some time to age. When dealing with an already blended perfume, it should not take too long to age. You could allow it to blend well over a week before using it.

Mixing Essential Oils in a Fresh Blend

While mixing essential oils in an existing blend is possible, it brings a lot of complications. On the other hand, mixing essential oils in a fresh blend is much easier and direct. As a matter of fact, all you need is the mixing formula to prepare your all-new perfume in a few steps. Here is the procedure to follow when mixing essential oils in a fresh blend.

Determine the essential oil to alcohol ratio: The first thing you should determine is your desired essential oil to alcohol ratio. This will depend on the type of perfume you wish to prepare. If you want to come up with a strongly scented perfume that may last the whole day on your skin, you will have to use less than 50% of alcohol. On the other hand, if you wish to prepare a premium perfume with a unique scent and moderated notes, you will have to use at least 65% alcohol. Whether you are using an already existing formula or you are trying to come up with your own unique scent, start by determining the alcohol to essential oil ratio. When calculating these ratios, also consider the need for additives such as fixatives and preservatives if necessary.

Determine your essential oil ratios: Once you have determined the alcohol to oil ratios, you also have to divide your essential oils accordingly. For amateur perfume makers, it is okay to combine your essential oils in equal measures. In other words, if your top note essential oil is 5 grams, you can also use a similar measure for middle notes and base notes. However, as you advance your skills, you should learn to play with the contents of the oil to attain a much-balanced scent. I will recommend using more oil for middle notes, followed by top notes and less oil for the base notes. The main reason why you should use more for top notes is that such essential oils evaporate much faster. If you wish your top notes to last a bit longer, use more quantity in your top notes. On the other hand, if you do not want your notes to last longer, increase the volume of middle notes and reduce the top notes.

Combine the ingredients in the right order: While determining the right ratios for your essential oils is important, it is also crucial to follow the right mixing order. As we move on to the next chapter, we are going to look at the order of mixing your essential oils to arrive at your preferred perfumes. The most important point to note for now is that you need to follow an orderly way whenever dealing with a unique recipe for a perfume.

Chapter 4: Perfume Recipes

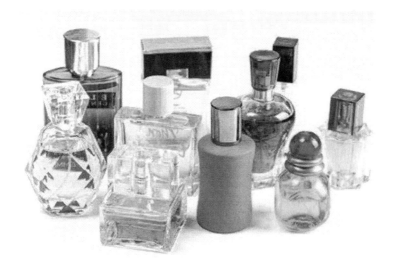

Now that we have looked at all the processes for preparing essential oils and the basic steps in preparing perfumes, it's time to make some perfumes. In this chapter, we are going to look at several recipes for homemade perfumes that you can easily prepare at home. We are going to make some liquid perfumes that you can spray on yourself at home and some solid perfumes.

Liquid Perfume Recipes

Liquid perfumes are the most common types of perfumes in the market. They are loved because of the ease of the application. With that said, liquid perfumes have a disadvantage of fast diffusion. In other words, they do not last on the skin or your clothes, as it is the case with solid perfumes. If you are interested in making some liquid perfumes at home, here are some formulas to help you.

Lavender Essential Oil Liquid Perfume

The first perfume we are going to prepare is inspired by the lavender essential oil. For this perfume, the lavender essential oil is going to form our top notes. Given that lavender is a well-pronounced smell and can readily be identified, it forms the perfect top note for our homemade essential oil perfume.

Ingredients:

Top Notes: 5 drops of lavender essential oil

Middle Notes: 9 drops of fractionated coconut oil

Base Notes: 5 drops tea tree essential oil

50 ml of 100 proof clear vodka

1 ml Phosphate buffered formalin (fixative)

Optional: bridging notes of your choice (I recommend vanilla for this recipe)

Directions:

1. In a bowl, add the fractionated coconut oil and warm gently to ensure that it is well liquified.

2. Now add the lavender essential oil and mix well with a small wooden stick. Cover the bowl with a plastic paper and let them stay undisturbed for about 30 minutes.

3. Now add the tea tree essential oil and mix well. Let them sit undisturbed for about 3 minutes. You may add in the optional bridging notes at this point.

4. Pour your clear vodka in a spray bottle to about the halfway mark. This means that you should use a spray bottle that can hold the

entire vodka and leave sufficient space above.

5. Now add the mixture of essential oils prepared earlier to the alcohol bottle and shake vigorously.

6. Let your perfume stay in the bottle overnight before tying it to feel its smell. If you feel the top note in your perfume when you spray, store it in a cool dark place to age. If you feel the smell of alcohol is too strong in your perfume, you may add a drop of the top notes to improve the smell.

7. Once you are satisfied with the smell of your perfume, add in the fixative and mix well. This will help prolong the time of smell on your skin or clothes.

The lavender inspired spray we have just prepared can last up to 6 hours on your skin. The top notes should vanish in 1 hour. From this point, you will experience the middle notes for about 2 hours and the base notes for about 3 hours. However, the effect of the notes also depends on your mixing formula, and the time taken to age. You may choose to make your top notes stronger by increasing their amount in your recipe.

Bay Rum Cologne Recipe

The second type of liquid perfume we are going to prepare is rum inspired cologne. Yes, we are going to use rum and Pimenta racemose bay oil to create our sweet-scented cologne. Here is the recipe:

Ingredients:

30ml of white rum

7 ml of witch hazel

Top Notes: 15 drops of Pimenta racemosa bay oil

Middle Notes: 5 drops clove essential oil and 10 drops of lime essential oil or 1 teaspoon of lime zest

Base Notes: 1/2 cinnamon stick or 1/2 teaspoon of cinnamon powder

Bridging Note: 1 tablespoon of vanilla extract

Directions:

1. Combine your rum with the witch hazel and water and mix well.

2. Once mixed, add in all the dry ingredients you will be using and gently bring all the ingredients to a simmer.

3. Once they simmer, remove from heat and cover the cooking pot well, until the liquid is fully cooled.

4. Transfer the liquid you have just prepared to the mason jar and tighten the lid. Store your perfume in a cool dark place for about 7 days.

5. After about 7 days of aging, remove the liquid from storage and filter out any solid matter with cheesecloth.

6. Now add the Pimenta racemosa bay essential oil to your perfume along with the other essential oils that you will be using. If you are adding fixatives, this is the time to add them to your perfume.

7. Transfer the perfume to a spray bottle and shake well, then spray to feel if it is has attained your desired scent.

If you are pleased with the scent, let the perfume settle in the bottle, then decant to remove any solid matter. Store your perfumes in a cool dark place and use it by spraying on your clothes or skin.

Note: Since this perfume is prepared by directly infusing fresh ingredients into the rum, it will have a very short shelf-life. To improve the shelf-life of your perfume, you may add preservatives such as glycerin or honey. The perfume should have a lifespan of about 3 months without the preservatives. The preservatives can prolong their lives to about 12 months or even more.

Rose Water Sweet Cologne

The other liquid perfume we are going to prepare is the rose water sweet cologne. Rose water on its own can be used as a basic perfume. However, we are going to introduce several ingredients that will help us develop a much stronger scent that is well balanced.

Ingredients:

Top Notes: 14 drops Rose flower essential oil

Middle Notes: 22 drops of lemongrass essential oil

Base Notes: 9 drops of neroli essential oil

Bridging Notes: 2 drops of lavender oil

85 ml of Rose Water

Instructions:

1. Combine all the essential oils above well in a small bowl until you feel the desired scent hit your nose. To ensure that you pick the right scent, cover your oils after mixing for a few minutes, and take a walk. When you come back, open the bowl and let the smell of the mixture hit your nose directly. You should remember that the scent will change over a few weeks as the contents start aging. You

should also note down this formula so that you can use it in the future in case you love the recipe.

2. Now add the rose water to your mixture and swirl to combine.

3. Transfer your rose water spray to a spray bottle and store it in a cool dark place for about 7 days.

4. After 7 days, spray your cologne to feel its smell. The smell will have matured to your preferred rose-scented cologne.

The cologne we have just prepared in this recipe can be spread on the skin or on clothes. However, you should first try with a small sample to determine whether it has any effect. If it causes itching on the skin or other allergic reactions, you will have to avoid it. Since we have used rose water in place of alcohol for this recipe, it has a very short shelf life. Make sure you use your cologne in 3 to 4 months. Thankfully, it can also be refrigerated for a much longer lifespan.

Peppermint Rose Water Cologne

The other rose water recipe involves the use of peppermint to come up with quick spray cologne. However, we are also going to use some alcohol in this recipe to give it a slightly longer shelf life and to improve the quality of our perfume.

Ingredients:

Top Notes: 12 drops of jasmine essential oil

Middle Notes: 8 drops of peppermint essential oil

Base Notes: 5 drops of cedarwood essential oil

20 ml of distilled water

20 ml of witch hazel

20 ml rose water

10 ml of 150 proof clear vodka of your choice

Directions:

1. Pour all the essential oils into a spray bottle and shake them well to combine.

2. Once well-combined, add in the rest of the liquid except for the alcohol and shake well to combine. Let them stay undisturbed for about 20 minutes.

3. If you will be using any fixatives, add them with the alcohol and shake well.

4. Store your perfume in a cool dark place for about 7 days, then take it out and test the spray. If it is up to your required standards, use it accordingly.

The perfume we have just prepared in this recipe can be sprayed on the skin and clothes. Make sure you use very clear alcohol if you will be spraying your clothes. The perfume has a shelf life of about 6 months, but it can be improved by adding preservatives such as glycerin.

Sweet Almond Essential Oil Perfume

The sweet almond essential oil is known for its medicinal purposes, but a few people know that it can actually be used in perfumery. The beauty of this oil is that it can be used to prepare all types of perfumes, including skin and hair sprays. Since the oil offers natural nutrients to your air, it provides the best option for those looking for a moisturizing hair spray. Here is the recipe for the sweet almond essential oil perfume that you can apply to your skin or hair.

Ingredients:

Top Notes: 5 drops of the sweet almond essential oil, and 5 drops of orchid essential oil

Middle Notes: 10 drops of clove essential oil

Base Notes: 10 drops of nutmeg essential oil.

Bridging Notes: 3 drops of lavender essential oil.

60ml of ethanol (any 100 proof or more clear vodka will work)

2 tablespoons of tap water

Directions:

1. Add the sweet almond oil into a spray bottle and add the rest of the essentials in the following order; base notes, middle notes, and finish with the top notes. This will mean that, although the sweet almond oil is one of the top notes, it will be the first in the bottle, while the other top notes will come last.

2. Once you are done, shake gently to mix before adding the bridge notes if you are using any.

3. Now add the entire alcohol to the bottle and shake the bottle for several minutes.

4. Keep the bottle in a cold place for about 48 hours to let the scent develop. Ideally, you can let the bottle stay up to 6 years for a much richer scent.

5. Once the scent develops to your desired level, add in 2 tablespoons of water and shake vigorously to mix.

6. Now, filter your perfume through cheesecloth to remove any solid matter and transfer it back to the spray bottle.

7. Store your perfume in a dark bottle away from the reach of direct sunlight.

The perfume we have just prepared can be sprayed directly to the skin or on clothes. Since it is made with some alcohol, it has a much longer lifespan than those prepared with non-alcoholic additives. However, you should add some preservatives if you want it to stay much longer.

Vanilla Lavender Spray

Lastly, let us look at how you can prepare some vanilla inspired lavender spray. In this perfume, we will have lavender as our top notes and vanilla as the middle notes. These sweet-smelling natural products will offer an amazing perfume that you can wear at any time of the day.

Ingredients:

Top Notes: 10 drops of lavender essential oil

Middle Notes: 12 drops of vanilla essential oil

Base Notes: cedarwood chips

30 ml 150 Proof clear vodka or higher

Directions:

1. Add the 10 ml of your clear vodka into a 1-ounce amber bottle

2. Add the vanilla and lavender essential oils in that order.

3. Cap your bottle and shake to mix well.

4. Add the cedar chips into your perfume and lock the bottle.

5. Let the perfume sit undisturbed in a cool dark place for at least 2 weeks. However, the perfume can be left to age for as much as 3 months for a better scent.

6. Once ready, filter out the cedar chips using cheesecloth and transfer about 10ml of the perfume to an atomized spray bottle for use.

Notes: The spray we have just prepared has a shelf-life of more than 2 years and will not need any preservatives. You should start by spraying it in the air to see if it has any effects on your respiratory system. You can then spray it on the back of your hand to see if it has any effect. If you love the smell, keep your perfume, and use it accordingly. This is one of the most durable body spray perfumes you can make at home due to the presence of cedarwood notes.

Solid Perfume Projects

Now that we are done with the liquid perfume recipes, let us look at some solid perfume recipes you can prepare at home. Solid perfumes are not any different from the liquid ones, except that they are prepared with some solid ingredients that make the final perfume solid. We can also prepare skin rub and lip balms.

Jojoba Oil Solid Perfume

The jojoba oil perfume is prepared with essential oils, just like the other perfumes in the recipes above. In this recipe, jojoba is combined with beeswax to ensure that the final product is solid. Here is the recipe.

Ingredients:

1 tablespoon of beeswax (you may also use petroleum jelly for the same purpose)

1 tablespoon of jojoba oil (this ingredient supplies essential vitamin E for your skin)

Top Notes: 2 ml of orchids essential oil

Middle Notes: 2 ml of lemongrass essential oil

Base Notes: 1 ml of sandalwood essential oil

Directions:

1. Add about 1 inch of water in a small saucepan and rest the jar containing the wax in the water. Bring the water in your saucepan to a boil, allowing the wax to melt completely.

2. Remove the wax from heat and add in all the essential oils in the order they are listed above. Stir gently with a thin mixing stick. If you do not stir the mixture immediately, it will start solidifying. When stirring, use a stick that is disposable to avoid having to deal with the tedious work of cleaning the wax later.

3. After mixing your ingredients well, pour the liquid mixture into the final container for storage.

4. After about 30 minutes, your perfume will have cooled down and ready to use. The perfume prepared here can be mixed with other skin applications such as lotions, jelly, lip balms, among others. You

can also directly apply the perfume to your skin. It is perfect for sweaty areas such as the underarms.

Coconut Oil Solid Perfume

The other type of solid perfume we are going to prepare is the coconut oil inspired perfume. This type of perfume is also made by blending various essential oils, except that we use beeswax to give it the solid form.

Ingredients:

1 teaspoon of coconut oil

Top Notes: 12 ml of rose essential oil

Middle Notes: 12ml of orchid essential oil

Base Notes: 10ml of oak wood essential oil

1 tablespoon of beeswax

2 tins, 15 mil in volume

Instructions:

1. Heat your almond oil over a double boiler; once it heats, add the wax pellets and continue heating until they are completely melted.

2. Once fully melted, stir with a wooden spoon to mix and remove from heat.

3. Add in the essential oils without following any particular order

4. These ingredients will make about 3 teaspoons of solid perfume, which can fill just about 2 x15 ml tins. If you are looking to make more perfume, double the recipe or triple it.

5. Once you are done, transfer your perfume to tins and let it stay unused for about 1 week.

6. Once ready, rub your perfume on your neck, wrist, or any part of your body. However, do not apply the perfume internally.

Notes: The beeswax we have used in this recipe is limited, and as a result, your perfume will be slightly liquid. The more wax you use, the more solid your perfume. You can use the perfume we have made to apply on the skin or a natural lip balm.

DIY Roll-on Perfume

Roll-ons are the signature perfume for those who do not enjoy colognes. We have prepared some cologne in the section above; you can also prepare some roll-ons at home and use them to reduce the body odor during the day.

Ingredients:

10ml essential oil bottle with a roller cap

1 tablespoon of fractionated coconut oil

2 tablespoons of sweet almond oil

Top Notes: 20 drops of jasmine essential oil

Middle Notes: Neroli essential oil

Base Notes: Geranium essential oil

Measuring cup

Instructions:

1. Add about 1 tablespoon of fractionated coconut oil into a measuring cup with a spout for pouring out.

2. Pour about 2 teaspoons of the sweet almond oil into the measuring cup.

3. Add in the jasmine essential oil and mix well.

4. Add in the neroli essential oil and mix well before adding the geranium essential oil.

5. Once you have mixed all the essential oils, your perfume should be creamy thick, although it will not be as solid. You can now transfer your perfume to a 10 ml glass bottle for the roller cap.

6. Place the roller ball on top of the bottle and apply some of the perfume on your palm to feel the scent. You may try improving the scent if you do not like it.

Basic Balm Recipe

The other solid perfume recipe we can prepare is the basic balm. Balms can be applied on the skin or on the lips. In this recipe, we are going to use cocoa butter and beeswax in combination with various essential oils. Here is the recipe.

Ingredients:

10 grams of beeswax

5 grams of cocoa butter

30 ml of coconut oil

10 ml of jasmine essential oil

10 ml of lemon essential oil

10 ml of cedarwood essential oil

Directions:

1. Combine all the oils and butter in a saucepan and warm them on slow heat while mixing until they are well mixed.

2. Transfer the melted oils and butter into a container, and it will harden over time.

3. After it hardens, just rub a finger into your balm and apply it to your skin.

4. This type of perfume works well for targeted areas such as the cuticles, the lips, and dry patches on the skin. It is also used as an under-eye treatment.

The reason I love this basic balm is that it can also help you develop a solid perfume that can be applied to the whole skin, lips, or skin salve by adding various essential oils.

Skin Salve Recipe from the Basic Balm Recipe

From the basic balm recipe above, we are going to develop a skin salve. You should start by developing a basic balm like the one above and use it to develop your salves.

Ingredients:

Basic balm recipe as prepared above

30 drops of any essential oil of your choice (you can also create an accord by blending various essential oils)

Directions:

1. Combine your essential oil mix with the balm in our recipe above over low heat and let them melt.

2. Once they are melted, feel the scent to see if it matches your desire. You may try adding in the top notes essential oils such as roses or lavender to give your perfume a more defined scent.

3. Add your salves in your container and store it for later use. The slave you have prepared here can now be applied to your lips and other parts for the skin. It can also be applied to pretty much your whole body, avoiding sensitive areas.

Note: The balm we have prepared in this recipe can stay for as long as a year without going bad. However, you should store your balm or perfume in a cold dark place, away from direct heat.

Natural Deodorant

The next solid perfume recipe we are going to look at is that of natural deodorant. The natural deodorant we prepare in this recipe is made by combining various essential oils with Shea butter. Here is the recipe.

Ingredients:

2 tablespoons of Shea butter

3 tablespoons of coconut oil

3 tablespoons of baking soda

2 tablespoons of arrowroot powder.

Top Note: 1 tablespoon of lavender essential oil

Middle Note: 1 tablespoon of clove essential oil

Base Note: 1 tablespoon of nutmeg essential oil

Instructions:

1. Place the Shea butter and coconut oil in a quart-size mason jar.

2. Place your mason jar in a small saucepan of water and heat the water until the butter and coconut oil are well melted and mixed.

3. Now remove the oils from heat and add in the other essential oils and mix further.

4. Add in the baking soda and arrowroot and mix well.

5. Transfer the mixture into a plastic container and store it in the fridge.

6. After about 12 hours of refrigeration, your deodorant should be ready for use. You can transfer it into an old deodorant stick for easier use.

Make sure you always store your deodorant in a cool dark place to prevent it from melting, especially during the summer.

Coconut Oil Salve Perfume

The other type of solid perfume we are going to prepare is the coconut oil salve perfume. The coconut oil salve is prepared by combining coconut oil with some essential oils and shea butter. Here is the recipe.

Ingredients:

3 tablespoons of coconut oil

2 tablespoons of Shea butter

2 tablespoons of arrowroot powder

5 ml Iris essential oils

5 ml Orchid essential oil

5 ml Cedarwood essential oil

Directions:

1. Melt the Shea butter and coconut oil in a double boiler as we have done in previous recipes.

2. Remove the butter from heat and add in the arrowroot powder.

3. Add in the essential oils according to the order they are presented in the ingredients.

4. Mix all the contents above well and transfer to a mason jar for storage.

The coconut oil salve prepared in this recipe can be applied to the skin directly or can be mixed with other oils and lotions applied on the skin.

Notes: If you choose to store your balm in a deodorant container, make sure you refrigerate it to avoid a situation where the deodorant melts and spoils.

Honeysuckle Fragrance Perfume

The honeysuckle fragrance oil perfume is made out of a solid perfume base with honeysuckle fragrance oil.

Ingredients:

2 ounces of solid perfume base

5 ounces of honeysuckle fragrance oil

1/4 teaspoon of rose gold mica

Instructions:

1. In a heat-safe saucepan, add the solid perfume base and melt in the microwave or on medium heat.

2. Measure about 5 ounces of heavenly honeysuckle fragrance oil in a glass container.

3. Add about 1/4 teaspoon of Rose Gold Mica to your fragrance oil above and combine well.

4. Now pour the fragrance and color mixture into the melted perfume above and mix well. The mica creates a light pink color in the perfume, which works perfectly for the lips. It can also make your skin shine if you will be applying on the skin. You may increase the amount of mica in your recipe if you want your balm to be much pronounced.

5. Pour the mixture into slippery lip tins and allow it to cool before using it.

With that, we have prepared our final perfume from natural ingredients. All of the perfume recipes in this book are entirely made out of natural ingredients, except for a few additives. If you follow the formulas provided accordingly, you will end up with amazing signature scents that will draw more people to you. While preparing liquid and solid perfumes is a tiresome job, the hard part becomes storing and preserving your perfumes. As we have already mentioned, these perfumes are prepared from natural ingredients. As you may already know, most natural ingredients are prone to going bad if they stay for too long. Thankfully, most essential oils have a very long shelf life. Even in that case, we still have to find appropriate ways of preserving our perfumes to ensure that they do not go bad when we still need them. Further, having a clear understanding of the storage needs of perfumes gives you an opportunity to divide the volumes of production. The perfumes that go bad faster should be produced in limited amounts to avoid unforeseen losses in the future.

How to Store Your Finished Perfume

In general, the storage of most homemade perfumes does not require any special tools. Perfumes made at home can be stored at room temperature and will retain their scent for a very long time. However, there are a few factors that count and determine the expected lifespan of the perfume after it has been produced. Some of the important factors to keep in mind about the preservation of perfumes include:

The volume of alcohol used in manufacturing the perfume: The first aspect that determines how long your perfume will stay on the shelf is the volume of alcohol used in the preparation. Alcohol is the best preservative you can use in your perfumes since it protects the perfume against bacterial attacks. Any perfume made with more than 50% of alcohol will have a shelf life of at least 1 year. For this period, you can store your perfume within room temperatures without having to worry about it going bad. However, if you reduce the volume of alcohol in your perfume, chances are that it might go bad earlier than a year. Other factors that may affect the shelf life of the perfume include the presence of water and fresh organic matter in your perfume.

The acidity level of the essential oils used: The other important factor to consider when dealing with perfumes is the acidity level of essential oils used. There are some perfumes we have prepared without necessarily blending alcohol in the recipe. Such recipes are much more vulnerable to bacterial attacks. However, if the essential oils used have a lower pH, chances are that they will last for a very long time. Low pH in essential oils means high acidity. Most essential oils that have a pH level lower than 6 can last up to 3 years on the shelf. However, given that we have to blend various types of essential oils to come up with our perfume, the blend will have a much shorter lifespan. If you have to use essential oils without other additives, you should expect your perfume to have a lifespan of at least 1 year. However, if you have added water or fresh mater to the essential oils, the lifespan might be reduced. I must mention that most perfumes made out of pure essential oil or essential oil and alcohol will last for as long as 3 years. However, since we are not sure the type of compounds you may choose to add to your essential oil, it is important to keep the shelf life to the lower end.

Presence of fresh components in the perfume: The other important aspect to keep in mind about the storage of your perfumes is the presence of fresh components. If you have used fresh components such as cinnamon powder, cedarwood, or any other component in your recipe, it will have a shorter shelf life. This gets even worse if your recipe does not contain any alcohol. A recipe that includes fresh compounds and alcohol should give you a shelf life of about 6 months. This means that if you are preparing any perfume that will contain fresh compounds, only produce a small amount that can be used within months. However, if your perfume does not contain any alcohol and contains fresh elements, its shelf-life might be as short as 48 hours in some cases. Check each of the recipes above to get a more accurate picture of the shelf life. For perfumes that have such a short lifespan, the best option is to refrigerate. This might give them a shelf life of up to a few weeks, if possible.

Usage of water in the recipe: The other important aspect to consider when thinking about storage is the presence of water in your recipe. Water is the ultimate ingredient needed to cause bacterial infection in most perfumes. The recipes we have prepared with water or rose water have a much shorter shelf life as compared to those that we have prepared with alcohol. In other words, if any perfume has water as a major element, you should store it very carefully to improve its shelf-life. Normally, we store such perfumes under refrigeration to give them a shelf-life of a few weeks or months.

Exposure to light and heat: The most important factor to keep in mind when it comes to the storage of perfumes is exposure to light and heat. As we have already seen, all our perfumes are prepared out of essential oils and other natural products. One of the biggest problems with essential oils is that they are very volatile. If they are exposed to heat or air, they evaporate. If they are exposed to heat in a closed bottle, they may not evaporate, but the structure of the oil may change. A change in the compound structure effectively means that the oil might lose its scent even if it is inside the bottle. This is the reason why I have given out instructions to store your perfumes in a dark bottle. If you want your essential oil perfume to have a long shelf life, ensure that it is kept away from direct light, heat, and open air. Store the perfumes in a cool dark place and only remove from storage once in a while. For perfumes that have a shelf life of up to 1 year, you can store yours in a dark closet. In this case, only pour a little perfume in a decorative bottle for regular use. Once it is finished, top it up from the main source to avoid direct exposure to light or air.

Possible use of preservatives: Lastly, the other factor to consider when it comes to the storage of your perfume is using preservatives. For some of our recipes, we have either used glycerin or honey as a natural preservative. I highly recommend the use of preservatives for perfumes that are made with fresh compounds. Fresh compounds are likely to lead to bacterial attacks on your perfume and reduce its shelf life. If your perfume has a shelf life of 48 hours or a few weeks, you can increase it by adding some preservatives. With that said, natural preservatives such as glycerin will not give your perfume a very long life. Some will just increase its shelf life by a few weeks or months.

With all that said, it is important to ensure that you store your perfumes in the correct manner. Make sure they are not exposed to heat or light. If you have used alcohol and essential oils in any perfume, protect it from direct heat and exposure to the sun.

Chapter 5: Bonus Perfume Making Tips

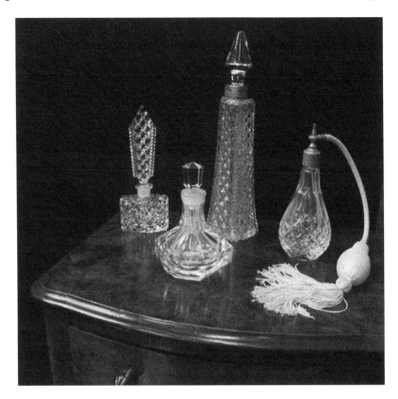

Now that you are done with preparing perfumes, let us look at some of the tips that can help you prepare your perfumes well. When preparing perfumes, there is a possibility that you will end up getting into problems along the way. We are going to look at the tips on how to handle any inconveniences and how to ensure that your perfume functions according to your preferences.

Troubleshooting Perfume Issues

There are many issues that could occur during the perfume-making process that will make your perfume-making process useless. Some of the issues that may occur and their possible solutions include:

Perfume does not last longer than an hour.

One of the common problems that perfume makers encounter is that perfumes vanish much quicker than anticipated. If you prepare a cologne that is intended to last at least 2 hours on the skin, you should expect it to have variations of a few minutes. Some perfumes may last longer, while others might last shorter. The only problem would be if the perfume only lasts a few minutes. If your perfume only lasts a few minutes, there are three possible causes. Probably, you have not added the base essential oil, or you have used too much alcohol. The other error could be that the middle notes and base notes used in the oils are highly volatile.

To ensure that your perfumes last for intended hours on your skin, you should make sure you use sufficient amounts of base notes. You may even add some base notes or middle notes to your perfume long after it has been prepared. The other option would be reducing the amount of alcohol used in the recipe. This would mean that you adjust some arrays of the recipe to ensure that the final outcome of the perfume-making process is a perfume that lasts on the skin. Lastly, you could try changing your middle notes to another essential oil. The middle notes are the essential oils that are second in the order of diffusion. Once the top notes diffuse and lose strength, the scent of the middle notes takes over. If you use essential oil that is very volatile for the middle notes, chances are that it will evaporate together with the first notes. This will consequently mean that your perfume loses strength much faster than anticipated.

Perfume stains my clothing.

The other common problem experienced in-home perfumery is a case where the perfume stains clothes. Perfume stains are usually caused by colored perfumes. If the perfume is prepared by adding fresh ingredients such as flowers or cinnamon sticks in your recipe, chances are that the perfume might stain your clothes. If you have prepared perfume with such fresh ingredients, do not spray it on white clothing. Further, perfumes that are prepared with colored vodka might also stain crystal white shirts. In case you use perfume that is colored and can possibly stain your clothes, do not spray it over your clothes. In such a case, you may spray the perfume on your skin instead of spraying on your clothes. When it comes to solid perfumes, you should never apply to your clothes under any condition. Most solid perfumes are designed for the skin and are not ideal for applying on any type of clothing.

Perfume does not spray.

The other possible trouble you might experience in perfumery is the failure of the perfume bottle to spray. There are various causes of failed perfume sprays. The first and most common cause for failure is the tubes being clogged by dirt. The second reason might be that the perfume bottle does not have a straw long enough to fetch the perfume. To deal with these issues, you have to first ensure that the perfume prepared is free of any solid matter. In case you have used some fresh matter in your perfumes, chances are that the perfume may retain some distillates. These distillates are likely to block the spray bottle, causing problems during spraying. To avoid such a situation, ensure that your perfumes are well filtered before transferring to the spray bottle. If you see some particles in your perfume, filter it several times with a filter paper to ensure that there are no large particles that may lead to spray issues. The other issue to sort out is the short perfume suction straw. For this purpose, just ensure that you purchase the best spray bottles for your project.

The perfume has gone rancid.

The other possible issue you might experience is the perfume going rancid. The perfumes we have prepared in the recipes above are made out of natural products. In other words, some of the compounds used in recipes can easily lead to rancidity. If you realize that your perfume is going rancid much faster than anticipated, chances are that you have made some errors. First, if the perfume is made with some water, ensure that you do not use too much water in the recipe. Water provides the best ground for the perfume to go rancid. Secondly, if the perfume is made with fresh ingredients, you should use a preservative. Natural preservatives such as glycerin can be used to help you deal with rancidity.

Perfume does not have a scent.

There are situations where you may prepare perfume, and it turns out without a clear scent. Though this is rare, it might happen if your perfume is exposed to too much heat or sunlight. After you prepare your perfume, ensure that you use the right storage approach to keep it scented. If the perfume is not stored appropriately, it might lose its scent over time. This is especially common in perfumes that are aged for a very long time. If you do not provide the right aging environment, the perfume might lose its scent due to prolonged exposure to air or heat.

Dealing with Allergens

While you may prepare the best perfume with some of our recipes, there is no guarantee that the perfume will be suitable for you. There are many people who experience allergic reactions to some perfumes.

Symptoms of Allergic Reaction

Some of the allergic reaction symptoms you might experience include:

Headaches: Headaches are among the most common allergic reactions to unique scents. Although most people do not associate headaches with the perfume, it is common for perfumes to cause headaches. If you apply the perfume and start experiencing a headache a few minutes later, you should know that it has a negative effect.

Nausea: The other common sign of an allergic reaction is nausea. If the perfume does not work well with your system, you may feel like vomiting or similar signs.

Skin Redness: The other common type of allergic reaction is skin redness. There are two main types of allergic reactions. You may either experience respiratory problems or skin reactions. The most common sign of skin-based allergic reaction is the redness of the skin. If you observe red spots on your skin after applying the perfume, you should stay away from it.

Skin Itching and Burning: Besides the redness of the skin, the other common symptom of an allergic reaction to perfume is itchiness. As a matter of fact, redness of the skin is often brought about by itchiness. If you start feeling itchy immediately after applying your perfume, do not scratch your skin. It will lead to blisters or redness of the skin.

Watery, Itchy, and Red Eyes: Besides respiratory and skin allergic reactions, you may also experience itchiness or watery eyes. Itchy eyes or watery eyes are as a result of the perfume affecting your eye cells internally. If you start dropping tears after applying the spray, chances are that you are being affected by the perfume you have just prepared.

Sneezing: The common symptom of respiratory problems when you use any perfume is sneezing. If you are reacting negatively to any perfume, you will feel an itching sensation in your nose accompanied by sneezing.

Runny Nose: If you feel an itching sensation or any sneezing, do not use your fingers to scratch your nose. If you start rubbing against your nose, you may aggravate some vessels and cause bleeding. It is common for some perfumes to cause nose bleeding on their own.

Breathing Difficulties: The other common respiratory symptom is difficulty in breathing. If you feel your mucus building up and some difficulty in breathing after using the perfume, chances are that it is contributing to your reaction.

Chest Tightness: The other common symptom of allergic reactions is chest tightness. If you happen to feel the chest getting tight after spraying the perfume, chances are that it is causing the reaction. You can try spraying the perfume at a later time to see if it is the one responsible for your reaction. If your reaction is being caused by the perfume, you will feel it again.

Worsened Asthma Symptoms: If you suffer from asthma, chances are that you may end up showing some symptoms after spraying the perfume. If the perfume causes an allergic reaction, it may lead to increased asthma symptoms.

Mitigating Allergy Symptoms

If you realize that you are experiencing the above allergic reactions, you may take some actions to prevent them.

Wear a Mask: If the allergic reactions you experience are respiratory, you can avoid them by wearing a mask when spraying.

In most cases, the perfume will only cause a reaction if it enters your nose during spraying. An N95 mask will stop about 95% of the perfume particles from penetrating into your nose. This way, you get to avoid allergic reactions since most triggers are stopped from entering the nose. The most common allergens are just small particles like pollen that may be found in the perfume. Using a mask can effectively reduce the effect of these particles if used in the right manner.

Spray-on Clothes: If the allergic reactions caused by the perfume affect your skin, you can avoid them by spraying on your clothes. In some people, the only allergic reactions experienced occur after the perfume gets in contact with the skin. If you are among such people, you can void the allergic reactions by spraying your perfume on your clothes. In this case, it is advisable to spray your closet to avoid the chances of the perfume dripping on your skin when you spray.

Modify the Perfume Formula: In some instances, the allergic reaction is due to one ingredient present in your perfume. If you can find out the ingredient causing the reaction, you could replace it in your formula and come up with a new perfume that is similar to the previous one. For instance, if it is the lavender top notes that are causing allergic reactions, you may replace them with a less allergic product. To determine the allergic product in your recipe, you may be forced to expose yourself to all the ingredients used in preparing the oil. This will show you the product that causes the allergic reaction so that you can get it out of your formula. If you realize that more than 1 ingredient is causing the reaction, you may have to do away with the entire formula.

Go Natural: Lastly and most importantly, if you realize that most perfumes cause allergic reactions, stick to natural ingredients. The main cause of allergic reactions in commercial perfumes is synthetic compounds. If you do not do well with most commercial perfumes, you can prepare all-natural perfume with fewer effects. Thankfully, most of the perfumes we have prepared in this book are natural. We have used naturally occurring ingredients such as essential oils, water, and some fresh organic matter. If you experience serious allergic reactions to any perfume prepared with such natural ingredients, you should avoid perfumes entirely.

FAQs about Perfumes

We have answered plenty of questions in regard to perfume preparation at home. However, there are still plenty of questions that some perfume users may want to get answered. Here are some of the frequently asked questions in regard to perfumes and the answers.

Q. Does my hair color and skin type affect which perfumes I'll like?

A: The short answer is yes; you should consider your hair color and skin type when preparing your perfumes at home. As we have already seen, there are some essential oils that are naturally good for hair while others are good for the skin. When preparing your perfume, you should consider whether it will be applied to the hair or skin. If you apply on the skin, choose an essential oil that offers value for the skin. At the same time, as to whether the perfume will be applied on the skin or hair determines the other ingredients you use in preparing it. Some ingredients such as mica we used in the solid perfumes are only helpful in perfumes that are applied to the skin. Mica adds color to your perfume and cannot be applied to the hair.

Q. How long will the perfume last on me?

A: The duration of the perfume on the skin depends on how much alcohol or essential oils you use. In most cases, perfume should last between 2 hours and 8 hours on the skin. Deodorant may last longer, depending on the percentage of the scented ingredients. With that said, there are many factors that determine whether your perfume will be durable or not. If you use too much alcohol in the perfume, it will not last long. If you use moderate amounts of alcohol and other ingredients, the alcohol is likely to last at least 5 hours.

Q. How can I make my perfume last longer on my skin?

A: If you want your perfume to last longer, you could make it stronger by increasing the essential oils used and reducing the volume of alcohol. Whether you will be blending your oils in water or oil, the final scent and its duration depend on the volume of the middle notes and base notes. On the other hand, if you do not want to increase the value of essential oils in your recipe, you could add fixatives to your perfume. Fixatives will make your perfume last longer, even if it has high alcohol content.

Q. What can I do if I am allergic to perfume?

A: We have already looked at the possible allergic reactions associated with perfumes. There are two main types of allergic reactions associated with perfumes. You can either suffer from respiratory allergies or skin allergies. Respiratory allergies include those that lead to the blockage of the breathing system. You may end up having difficulty breathing, itchiness in your nose, nose bleeding, among other effects. If you are allergic to perfumes in terms of the respiratory system, you may either wear a mask when using your perfume or avoid using it entirely. On the other hand, you should spray your perfume on your clothes if you experience allergic reactions on your skin.

Q. What is a fragrance note?

A: Fragrance notes refer to a single compound in accord of a perfume. For instance, the scent of lavender in a perfume can be referred to as a note. Notes are divided into top, middle and base notes. The notes must be combined to offer the full scent of the perfume. Notes can either be extracted from natural compounds or can be manufactured through a synthetic process. The synthetic manufacturing process may lead to unique scents that are not readily available in nature.

Q. What do top, middle, and base notes mean?

A: Top notes represent the scents that are felt first when you get in contact with perfume. For instance, you may instantly feel a rose flower scent when you spray a certain perfume. Top notes are usually made out of highly volatile compounds, such that they only last for a few hours or minutes. The middle notes are scent compounds that are experienced after the top notes fade away. Although middle notes diffuse fast in the atmosphere, they are much slower as compared to the top notes. Lastly, base notes are the scent compounds that are experienced last on the skin after spraying the perfume. Base notes are usually made from natural compounds such as wood or musk. Due to the different notes, the scent experienced when you spray perfume changes with time. If the perfume has lavender top notes, rosemary middle notes, and cedarwood base notes, you will start by experiencing the top notes, followed by middle and base notes later.

Q. Is natural perfume the best?

A: Most people assume that natural perfumes are much better than artificial ones. While there are pros and cons to each type of perfume, natural perfumes are still a few steps behind artificial ones. Artificial perfumes are ideal since they have a diversity of scent. Most artificial perfumes use synthetic scents that are not easily found in nature. If you are looking to prepare a premium quality perfume, you should be willing to compromise some aspects of your natural ingredients and include artificial ingredients to make your perfume better. With that said, artificial perfumes have the disadvantage of causing allergic reactions in most people. If you have experienced allergic reactions with many brands of perfume, you can try preparing an all-natural perfume to feel the difference.

Q. What kind of ingredients are found in perfume?

A: There are many ingredients available in perfumes. Some perfumes are made up of purely synthetic compounds, while others are made up of diverse ingredients. You may choose to prepare your perfume with synthetic compounds or all-natural compounds. For most of the perfumes on our list, we have used all-natural ingredients, except for a few recipes. The best natural ingredients for your recipes include essential oils and alcohol. The essential oils are combined in a specific ratio and mixed with alcohol to offer the final desired scent. Whether you love synthetic or natural perfumes, you have both options at your disposal. However, you must first consider the pros and cons of synthetic versus artificial perfumes.

Tips and Tricks When Crafting Perfume

When making perfumes at home, there are several challenges that are experienced. Among the most common challenges include the perfume losing its scent and the perfume scent not lasting long, among others. We have looked at some of the common issues that are likely to occur when preparing perfumes at home. Further, there are some problems that a home perfume crafter might experience. For instance, if you have to make perfume from 100% natural ingredients, you might go through plenty of problems trying to find the best essential oils for your project. Thankfully, I have some tips and tricks that will help make your work easier and your perfume more effective. Here are some tips that will help you make your work effective.

1. Purchasing essential oils will save you time: While the book outlines the ways you can prepare your essential oils from scratch, it is sometimes better to purchase the essential oils than preparing them at home. You do not have to purchase all the essential oils needed in your recipe. However, you will save much time if you choose to purchase essential oils rather than preparing yours. Further, commercially produced essential oils are purer and contain fewer additives. They have a much stronger scent and are the best option for any person looking to prepare perfumes at home.

2. Add Petroleum Jelly on Pulse Points: The other common problem that is experienced by most people preparing perfumes at home is the inability of perfumes to retain scent for longer. While you might come up with the perfect blend of essential oils, the perfume might lose its sweet scent in a very short time. If you are experiencing such a problem, you can use petroleum jelly to retain the scent much longer. The ointment in the jelly can be used to hold the fragrance much longer. Just mix a portion of your perfume with some petroleum jelly and apply it on your neck, hands, and other parts of the body. However, if you have to use petroleum jelly to retain the scent of your perfume, choose one that is not scented. Some petroleum jelly products come with a very strong scent that may mess up with the smell of your perfume entirely.

3. Spray Your Hairbrush: There are those who prepare perfumes at home for the purpose of spraying the hair. Hair sprays can serve many purposes. The perfume can be used to moisturize the hair, to feed the hair with vitamins, or to give the hair a good smell. Whichever your purpose of preparing your perfume, you should ensure that it does not cause more harm to your hair. When you prepare your perfume with alcohol, it will likely lead to dehydration.

In most cases, we prepare hair perfumes with very little alcohol. Ensure that you use hydrating essential oils such as jojoba oil as part of the recipe for hair sprays. With that said, if you happen to use some alcohol in your recipe, you can reduce the dehydration it causes by spraying it on the brush. Instead of spraying the perfume to your hair directly, spray it on your hairbrush then use the brush to comb your hair. This way, the alcohol in the perfume evaporates and leaves you with the sweet-smelling essential oils to apply on your hair.

4. Don't Store It in the Bathroom: Humidity and dampness do not work well with perfumes. When you prepare perfumes at home, ensure that your ingredients and finished products are not stored in the bathroom or anywhere damp. If you store your perfume in a damp place such as the bathroom, it will likely break down and lose its scent. This is the reason why most people complain about their perfumes, losing scent after some time. It is important that you store your finished products in a cool, dry place for longer shelf life.

5. Moisturize: For you to retain the perfume on your skin much longer, it is recommended that you moisturize. Perfumes lose their scent much faster when they are applied to dry skin as compared to a moisturized one. This applies to all types of perfumes, including the store-bought commercial ones. After preparing your perfume at home, you should ensure that it is used correctly to last as desired. There are many ways of moisturizing skin just before applying the perfume. You may either apply some petroleum jelly or lotion on your skin to moisturize it. Spray your perfume on top of the lotion or petroleum jelly to retain it much longer.

6. Apply it at the Right Time: applying the perfume at the wrong time might also be problematic. You may end up thinking that you have prepared the wrong perfume while it is your timing that is wrong. After preparing your perfume and ensuring that it meets your quality needs, you should try it on. If you spray your perfume on moisturized skin, it will stay much longer. However, if you spray in one of your skin and wear your clothes immediately, chances are that the clothes will rub the spray away. Most people have often asked whether you should wear perfume before clothes or the other way round. The answer is simple, if you are spraying on the skin, spray it first, give it a few minutes to dry, then wear your clothes. On the other hand, if you are wearing it on your clothes, put on the clothes first before spraying perfume.

7. Avoid Friction: The top notes of any perfume will vanish away much faster than the middle and base notes. The case gets even worse if the perfume is exposed to friction. After spraying your perfume on your body, ensure that there is no friction. For instance, if you spray the perfume on your wrists, do not rub them against each other. Rubbing any part of your body after applying the perfume will most likely lead to the perfume vanishing away much faster.

8. Mix Perfume with Lotion and Petroleum Jelly: Most people often end up wasting precious perfume by disposing of the perfume bottle once a small amount is left at the bottom. Do not waste any perfume that you can use. If you have undergone the hard process of extracting essential oils, you should know how valuable perfumes are. In my case, I usually mix any leftover perfumes or essential oils with my lotion and petroleum jelly. Mixing perfumes with lotions or petroleum jelly will help you utilize the perfume to the last drop. Further, lotions have preservatives that may help prolong the shelf life of your perfume. If you realize that your perfume is just about to start losing its scent or is at the risk of going bad, mix it with your regular perfume and use it as you would use on any other day.

9. The Less Essential Oils, the Better: One tip about making perfumes I wish I learned earlier is that more essential oil is not the best solution. As a matter of fact, you should try to reduce the amount of essential oils used in your project as much as possible. When we are making perfumes at home, we are trying to achieve a certain type of perfume. From the sections above, we've looked at the common types of perfume, including body sprays such as Eau de Cologne or Eau de Toilette. We have also looked at deodorants and other types of perfumes. One thing that stands out is that most of the premium perfumes do not contain as many essential oils. Most premium perfumes are at least 65% alcohol. In other words, if you want to attain a more balanced and sweet-smelling perfume, you will have to do away with too many essential oils and try introducing other components. Most importantly, you should always ensure that you use more alcohol in your perfumes to attain the scent you are going for.

10. Carry Around Cotton Balls: It is common for most people to carry around perfumes in their bags to freshen up once the perfume scent fades away. There are various ways of dealing with this problem. You could either use fixatives to improve the duration of your perfume, or you could use the options of petroleum jelly discussed above. However, if you realize that your perfume still fades away much faster even after applying it over petroleum jelly or lotion, you can use cotton balls to carry along with some perfume. Instead of carrying around heavy bottles of perfume everywhere you go, just dip some cotton balls in the perfume and bring them along. The cotton balls will retain the sweet perfume scent much longer and will remain wet as long as they are in your bag. Pat the cotton balls in your armpits or any part of the body that you want to smell fresh.

11. Don't Shake Your Perfume: Perfumes are not supposed to be shaken every time you use them. If you shake your perfume regularly, chances are that some air might get in. As we have discussed above, perfumes will lose their scent if they are exposed to air. The more you shake your perfume, the more you expose it to air. Exposing your perfume to air means that it will lose its smell long before you use it. To avoid such a case, ensure that you do not shake your perfume vigorously when using it.

12. Keep the Box: Lastly and most importantly, the storage of perfumes should be away from the reach of light. We have already discussed the effect that heat and light may have on your perfume. Even if you choose to store your perfume in a transparent bottle, always ensure that the bottle is kept inside a box or a cabinet. If you do not have a perfume box at your disposal, just purchase any type of box and use it to store your perfume. In my case, I use gift boxes to store my perfumes in small amounts. You may also use old perfume bottles and boxes to store your homemade perfumes so that they do not lose their scent. If you expose your perfumes or even essential oils to direct light, they will lose their scent.

Precautions and Mistakes to Avoid

While making perfume might be a straightforward process, there are many people who make mistakes that could be costly. Perfumes should not be prepared by a person who doesn't understand the type of ingredients being used. If you are not careful, the entire process may lead to injuries and losses. Some of the precautionary measure and mistakes you should consider when making perfumes include:

1. Do not prepare your perfumes next to open flame: The first mistake that most people make is preparing perfumes next to open flames. When preparing perfumes, you should remember that all the ingredients are highly flammable. Both alcohol and essential oils are very flammable. If you open these ingredients next to open fire, you risk starting a fire that might lead to devastating losses. To avoid burning your house down, ensure that you prepare your perfumes away from open flames. If any of the ingredients need heating, heat them in a closed saucepan on very low heat. Stay vigilant throughout the process to avoid a case where the heat causes a fire outbreak in your home.

2. Wear protective gear when preparing perfumes: The other mistake that most people make is forgetting to wear protective gear. Wearing protective gear is a very important part of perfumery. One of the factors to keep in mind is that some essential oils might lead to allergic reactions. Before you start preparing your perfume, make sure you wear a face mask, hand gloves, and a pair of sunglasses. The gloves will protect your hands from getting in direct contact with the oils. As mentioned, the essential oils are likely to lead to allergic reactions on the skin. Secondly, the face mask will protect your respiratory system from possible respiratory reactions. The respiratory system can be affected by some of the oils and other ingredients used in the process. Lastly, the sunglasses help protect your eyes from any perfume, alcohol, or essential oils that may splash over. If perfumes splash over, they may affect your eyes and cause long-term vision problems.

3. Do not mix your kitchen utensils with perfumery tools: The other mistake that most people make is combining kitchen utensils with perfumery tools. While it is okay to borrow some of your kitchen tools for your perfumery work, you should not mix them without drawing lines. If you choose to pick any tool from your kitchen for your project, do not take it back to the kitchen until you are done with the project and thoroughly cleaned all the utensils. Perfumes are made using many ingredients, some of which might be harmful to the human body when ingested. Even some of the essential oils may lead to stomach problems or other complications if mixed with foods. For this reason, stick to using your perfumery tools that are different from kitchen ones.

4. Don't forget to label all the ingredients and tools: The reason why most people end up mixing ingredients and tools is a failure to label. This is a big mistake that you must avoid if you wish to have a successful perfumery project. When buying your tools and materials, make sure you buy a labeling tape that will help you distinguish ingredients in your work station. When labeling, make sure you indicate the name of every item in your work station, its purpose, and the date of labeling. This way, you can keep track of perfume aging periods. If you do not label perfume bottles, you may get confused and end up missing the ideal aging period. You may also mix essential oils and end up with perfumes that are not interesting to smell.

5. Storage of all your tools and ingredients matters: The storage of tools, ingredients, and the final product is very important. We have already looked at how you are supposed to store your essential oils, fresh plant extracts, and perfumes. If you do not follow the right storage protocols, all your ingredients will get spoiled even before you start preparing the perfumes. Essential oils are particularly very unstable when exposed to heat, air, and light. Make sure you store such ingredients in the right manner as stipulated above so that you can prepare a perfume that meets your requirements.

6. Keep perfumes and ingredients away from children: Lastly, children can be fun to have around, but they can also be destructive. If you will be doing your perfumery work in a place where children are allowed to access, you need to find a way of storing your ingredients from their reach. For instance, if you are working from your kitchen, make sure that all your essential oils, alcohol, and fixatives are stored in an elevated cabinet. Further, have a lock on your cabinet to avoid a situation where kids end up drinking raw ingredients. However, the best way to ensure that children do not mess up with your ingredients is by storing them in a room where they cannot access.

Conclusion

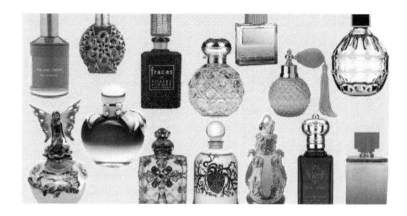

Congratulations on reading this book to the end, and thank you. I believe that you have learned a lot of new skills about perfumery that you did not know. You have probably mastered a few perfume recipes that you are about to get started with. However, before you even start preparing perfumes at home, I would recommend reading the book one more time. Reading this book over again should open your eyes to perfumery in a clearer manner.

You have now gotten a rough idea of what you need and how to go about every process of perfume making. However, if you really want to make the best perfumes out there, you need to read the book one more time with a practical approach. In your second reading, make sure you take action at every step where you are required to. Once you come to the section about tools, ensure that you go out and shop for all the tools you need. Get everything you need in a step by step approach until you are ready to start your projects.

This book takes a practical approach, and every person who wishes to benefit from it must be practical. I have divided the book into three main practical sections and 1 informational section. To help you benefit from the book the most, we start off with the informational section. I will highly recommend reading all the information provided in the book so that you can get the practical aspects well. In the informational chapters, we mainly look at the general information about perfumes. For instance, the first chapter covers the terminologies you should expect in the book. This chapter offers a clear view of what the book should contain. Without reading the first chapter, you may not know the meaning of terms such as accord, notes, scent, perfume, etc. These terms are very vital in the practical steps of developing perfumes from scratch.

In the practical sections of the book, we start by looking at the tools we will need for the entire project. We look at the materials needed to acquire essential oils, plant matter extracts such as tinctures, and infusions for the project. After determining the tools and materials, we look at the process that can help us extract essential oils, tinctures, infusions, and other extracts from plants. Most of our recipes mainly involve naturally occurring scents that can be extracted from plants and animals.

In the second section of our practical guide, we look at the step by step process of preparing liquid perfumes. The book elaborates and outlines the basic steps involved in perfume preparation. The book further introduces you to practical scent development. We show you how to come up with a unique scent, how to add essential oils to an existing scent, and how to improve the duration of the particular scent. We then move on to preparing unique perfumes based on customized recipes. All the perfumes we have prepared are made out of natural ingredients with some additions such as preservatives and fixatives. We show you how to prepare both liquid and solid perfumes that can be applied at home.

Finally, crown up the book by looking at some precautionary measures you should take and the mistakes you should avoid. We also look at special tips that will help you prepare the best perfumes and how to wear your perfume. Some people prepare very good perfumes but fail to understand the best way on how to wear them. This book shows you the best way to wear perfume and ensure that it lasts on your body.

If you are a fan of perfumes or looking for a way to enjoy life by trying out various types of perfumes, this book is for you. This book will help you to come up with new unique scents that will add some flavor to your life. Once you learn how to prepare your first few perfumes, you can go ahead and try your own recipes. Good luck with your perfumery and have fun.

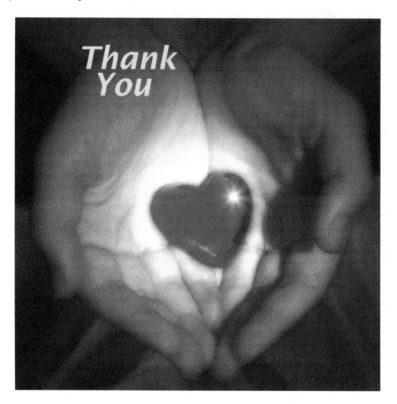

Would you please consider leaving a review where you purchased this book? Online reviews help me reach a wider audience. Thank you in advance!

Made in the USA
Columbia, SC
25 October 2024

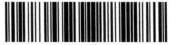